Professional Practice
for Podiatric Medicine

Edited by
Catherine Hayes

Professional Practice for Podiatric Medicine
Dr Catherine Hayes

ISBN: 978-1-905539-82-6

First published 2013

British Library Cataloguing in Publication Data
A catalogue record for this book is available from the British Library

Notice

Clinical practice and medical knowledge constantly evolve. Standard safety precautions must be followed, but, as knowledge is broadened by research, changes in practice, treatment and drug therapy may become necessary or appropriate. Readers must check the most current product information provided by the manufacturer of each drug to be administered and verify the dosages and correct administration, as well as contraindications. It is the responsibility of the practitioner, utilising the experience and knowledge of the patient, to determine dosages and the best treatment for each individual patient. Any brands mentioned in this book are as examples only and are not endorsed by the publisher. Neither the publisher nor the authors assume any liability for any injury and/or damage to persons or property arising from this publication.

To contact M&K Publishing write to:
M&K Update Ltd · The Old Bakery · St. John's Street
Keswick · Cumbria CA12 5AS
Tel: 01768 773030 · Fax: 01768 781099
publishing@mkupdate.co.uk
www.mkupdate.co.uk

Designed and typeset by Mary Blood
Printed in England by H&H Reeds, Penrith

Professional Practice
for Podiatric Medicine

Other books from M&K include:

A Guide to Research for Podiatrists
ISBN: 9781905539413

A Pre-Reader for the Foundation Degree in Health and Social Care Practice
ISBN: 9781905539680

Research Issues in Health and Social Care
ISBN: 9781905539208

Valuing People with a Learning Disability
ISBN: 9781905539666

Timely Discharge from Hospital
ISBN: 9781905539550

Contents

With much love for Charlotte, Elizabeth and Juliette Hayes

About the Author

Since qualifying in Podiatric Medicine at The Durham School of Podiatric Medicine in 1992 Catherine Hayes has worked within the National Health Service and in Private Practice before becoming a full time academic in the Department of Pharmacy Health and Wellbeing at the University of Sunderland, where she is currently Programme Leader for postgraduate provision and a director of studies for doctoral students.

Acknowledgements

Thanks firstly to the individual authors who contributed to this book, all of whom I have the great privilege of also being able to call my friends; I hope this will be the first of many opportunities to work together. Finally, a huge thank you to all of my friends and colleagues at the University of Sunderland and to the wider circle of podiatrists I have had the pleasure of working over the last twenty years in podiatric medicine.

Preface

Professional practice for podiatric practitioners is not a new phenomenon; it has dominated the focus of educational discussion and debate on how best the scope and parameters of podiatric medicine can be developed for the majority of two decades. Much has focused on how traditional academic theoretical perspectives on professionalism can be translated into applied clinical practice at the front line of patient assessment, diagnosis and management. Written by a selection of dedicated practitioners and educators from the field of healthcare generally and podiatric medicine specifically, the overall aims of this book are to:

- raise an awareness of professional practice for podiatric practitioners through an engagement with the core clinical, intellectual and analytical skills required for healthcare generally and podiatric practice specifically;
- provide a resource for members of the podiatric practitioner community, which addresses the fundamental contributory factors of professional practice in key areas such as professional identity, clinical professional practice, management and leadership alongside education and continuing professional development;
- develop an approach which enhances the healthcare practitioner's ability to engage with and build capacity between professions in an inter-disciplinary and multi-disciplinary approach to high quality healthcare provision.

Initial qualification within a particular profession is now deemed a foundation for the building of a solid, continuing professional development portfolio, which may subsequently become part of an evidence base for individual accountability and governance by professional regulatory bodies. This book aims to address how we can best synthesise the evidence base for the provision of care rooted in the best published literature to date from specific fields of academic research.

After a significant period of professionalisation podiatric medicine is now a discipline which still engages heavily in debate around the concept of its own professional identity and the contextual framework for practice. This book offers an insight into how this might be sociologically framed as well as practically executed.

Principles of leadership and management which impact on individual career progression pathways and personal development opportunities within healthcare

are discussed alongside the processes of appraisal, work loading and continuing professional development, which continue to shape the future of the profession as a whole through individual commitment to podiatric medicine.

Our sustained contribution to the concept of patient-centred care and our unique contribution to the allied healthcare professional arena have ensured that our own levels of clinical professional practice have never before been under closer scrutiny. Our commitment to its ongoing progression is therefore fundamental to our credibility as a profession.

Chapter One

Professional Identity –
Who do we think we are?

Judith Barbaro-Brown

Framing Professional Identity

In podiatry, as in all healthcare professions, the development of a professional identity is an essential part of learning about what it is to be 'a podiatrist'. For many practitioners this is a process which begins in the early years of clinical education and experience, and may be highly influenced by the attitudes and perceptions of those involved in helping the student along the educational pathway. The student is socialised into the profession by the development of a notion of what that profession is, and this continues throughout formal education and on into professional practice. Additionally, exposure to clinical situations and other healthcare professionals help students and practitioners learn about the roles of other professions, as well as the differences between them, contributing to an appreciation of what it is to be a 'professional', with the attitudes, behaviours, and perceptions that are attached to this. However, along with the benefits gained by this exposure come potential problems in that it is not only positive attributes which can be passed on. These detrimental influences may not only come from other professionals, but also from wider society and the media. Negative stereotypes relating to other professions and a poor perception of one's own profession can be highly significant, and lead to dissonant views relating to inter-professional and group working. It is the aim of this chapter to examine the development of identity in terms of the social and professional self, and reflect on how we, as professionals, can enable the promotion of positive and cohesive identities which allow us to contribute effectively to team-working, whilst appreciating the underlying issues which can interfere with a collaborative, inter-professional approach.

Social Identity and Identity Development

Professional identity can be seen as an extension of social group identity, a group being defined as a number of people who perceive themselves in terms of shared knowledge, skills, or attributes, which sets them apart and distinguishes them from other people (Hogg, 2006, p. 111). Professional identity involves group interactions in the workplace and more specifically relates to how individuals compare and differentiate themselves from other professional groups. Being a member of a group is a pivotal principal of social identity theory, which addresses phenomena such as in-group and out-group behaviour, stereotyping, discrimination, conformity, prejudice, leadership, and cohesiveness (Helmich *et al.*, 2010).

Social Identity Theory

Social Identity Theory (SIT) was initially described by Henri Tajfel and John Turner (Tajfel & Turner, 1979), and was originally founded on their attempts to explain inter-group reactions and conflict (Hogg & Vaughan, 2005 p.411). It is based on the assumption that society is categorised into different social groups that are seen to have differing levels of status and power in relation to each other. Being a member of one of these groups gives an individual a social identity, which defines that individual in terms of their behaviours and attributes. In this way, members of different social groups develop an understanding of the perceived behaviours and characteristics of members from other social groups. Related behaviours to this are stereotyping, prejudice, in-group and out-group perceptions, and group cohesiveness.

> A pivotal assumption of SIT is that in-group bias is wholly motivated by the wish to have one's group valued highly, and therefore to see oneself in a positive light.
>
> *(Brown, 2000)*

An individual can have numerous social identities depending on the number of social groups to which they feel aligned. These groups can sit within any aspect of society, from personal and reciprocal relationships (mother/daughter), to employment (teacher, cleaner, nurse), activity (footballer, cyclist, artist, Scout), ethnicity (Afro-Caribbean, South Asian, European), religion (Christian, Muslim, Hindu), or locality (Glaswegian, Cockney, Parisian).

Self-Categorisation Theory

Since SIT was first put forward there has been a great deal of further development from which other theories have emerged, and perhaps the most significant of these was by Turner *et al.*, known as Self-Categorisation Theory (Turner, 1996), with the proposition that the actual process of categorising oneself as a member of a group produces social identity, and from this, group and intergroup behaviours are developed. In essence, social identity is the definition of 'self' in regard to the groups to which one belongs, and it may be more appropriate to view this in terms of the social identity perspective (Hogg & Vaughan, 2005, p. 408).

Self-Categorisation Theory (SCT) states that the perception a person has of themself varies, and each person has the capacity to hold multiple self-concepts (social identities), and therefore belong to a number of categories, although at a given time only one of these self-concepts is salient. However, this does not imply that this is always the dominant self-concept, but that depending on the circumstances, different self-concepts can be activated (Mackie & Smith, 1998; Salzarulo, 2004). The category to which an individual assigns him or her self at any given moment is termed the self-category, or in-group. It is the fundamental hypothesis of Self-Categorisation Theory that as we group the individuals around us into subsets, we identify ourselves with the group whose membership shows the most similarity to ourselves (Oakes *et al.*, 1991).

Categorisation, Prototypes and Depersonalisation

The practice of categorisation (the clustering of people, objects, ideas, and/or events into meaningful groups) represents a very basic step in human judgement and perception, allowing an individual to process information rapidly and instinctively (Brewer, 2003). Categorisation forms the basis for identification of groups, and is a fundamental part of the study of how group relationships develop. Much of the early work in identifying the characteristics of categorisation was carried out by Gordon Allport in the early 1950s, from which he developed a model which stated that there were five important features of categorisation (Allport, 1979):

1. It forms large classes or clusters.
2. It assimilates as much information as possible into the cluster.
3. It enables rapid identification of a related object.
4. All members of the category are imbued with the same ideas and emotions.
5. Categories are based on existing differences between characteristics of objects or people.

Depending on the perception of the viewer, categorising another individual into a social group classifies that individual as being part of an in-group (to which the viewer also belongs) or an out-group (of which the viewer is a non-member), and therefore is subject to irrational reasoning. Allport recognised this, and stated therefore that social categorisation was often less than rational and frequently based on personal beliefs about social groups rather than actual evidence of group differences (Allport, 1979). In essence, it was at the mercy of personal bias and opinion.

A further step on from categorisation is the recognition that there is a tendency for exaggeration of the extent of differences between groups. Once a group has been identified, a prototype group member is represented, which consists of a group of attributes which distinguishes this group's members from another's. The prototype conforms to the **metacontrast principle** in that the average differences between members of the in-group are less than the average differences between the in-group and out-group members (Turner, 1996), which in turn accentuates **group entitativity – the property of the group that makes it appear different, distinct, and coherent** (Lickel *et al.*, 2000). The prototype is not a typical or average group member, but is more of the 'ideal' group member, embodying all the characteristics that would be associated with group membership, even if no single group member displayed all of the characteristics. In essence, the prototype is the context-dependent, cognitive representation of the group (Hogg & Vaughan, 2005, pp. 409).

> As an illustration of the metacontrast principle and entitativity, Hopkins and Moore (2001) looked at national group perceptions, and found that Scots had a clear perception of the differences between themselves and English people, but this amount of perceived difference between Scots and English reduced when comparing themselves to continental European groups such as Germans, i.e. the Scots were different to the English, but had more in common with English people than with German people.

This process of categorising people results in the depersonalisation of the individual, where they are perceived as a group member rather than an individual with their own views and idiosyncrasies. There is the tendency to project the group prototype on to the individual, thereby enhancing the perception of them as typical group members, holding standardised group values, and exhibiting standardised behaviours – known as stereotyping. This also occurs in the re-definition of the self (self-stereotyping), and consequently individuals begin to act in terms of their group identity rather than their personal identity (Tajfel & Turner, 1986). Once this group identity is salient, the individual looks for a positive evaluation of the group. From an intra-group perspective, this leads to cohesion and co-operative behaviour, whilst from an inter-group perspective, the in-group membership wish to feel superior to relevant out-groups (Voci, 2006). The resulting outcome in group behaviour is the development of **in-group bias**, or **ethnocentrism** (showing a preference for all aspects of the in-group relative to other groups). This process of depersonalisation appears to be the basis for the development of group cohesiveness, co-operation, trust, positive regard, and in-group favouritism (Hewstone *et al.*, 2002, Turner, 1996, Oakes *et al.*, 1991).

Salience

> Salience, in this context, refers to the current, psychologically significant persona of the individual within a specific social group or category, and the alteration of behaviour to act as a group member rather than an individual.

How an individual makes the decision about salient group membership is thought to depend on two factors – accessibility and fit (Bruner, 1957). **Accessibility** refers to how ready an individual is to recognise a category as being a distinct social group, e.g., gender, profession, political party, either because they are easily recognised from regular interaction (referred to as being chronically accessible), or because they appear obvious to the social situation (they are situationally accessible). Accessibility will depend on the current purpose and goal of the individual, together with how likely the individual is to encounter that category. For example, awareness of a support group for carers once one becomes a carer for a spouse or relative – the more the individual identifies with the role and the greater the recognition of the characteristics of a carer, then the more distinct and defined the requirements for that group's membership become, and the more likely it is that the individual will align themselves with the group.

Fit refers to the congruency between the category and the situation of the individual, i.e. how ready they are to see themselves as a group member. If a categorisation fits in the sense that it provides a valid reason for differences or similarities between people, then it is said to have structural fit, sometimes known as comparative fit. If the category also explains satisfactorily why people are behaving in particular ways, then it is said to have normative fit. If the category does not provide a good fit, i.e. similarities and differences do not correspond to the viewer's perception, then it is normal for the individual to work their way through a number of different accessible categories until one with the best fit is identified (Hogg, 2006, pp. 119). Bruner suggests that if two categories are equally accessible, then that with the best fit will become salient. If both categories have equally good fit, then the more familiar (accessible) category will become salient.

Motivation in Social Identity

Self-enhancement and uncertainty reduction appear to be the two processes which underlie the motivation to develop social identity. Individuals recognise that groups view each other in terms of relative status and prestige, and that within the social context some groups are viewed as being generally more prestigious and of higher status. Relationships between groups are frequently characterised by competition for collective high esteem, and to be different from other groups in terms of favourability. This positive inter-group distinctiveness allows group members to feel good about themselves by maximising the differences by which their group is superior to other groups.

Self-enhancement

The belief that one's own group is superior to another group is known as positive distinctiveness and is a feature of self-enhancement. Group members promote and protect this ethnocentric approach because this positive social identity attaches to the individual, thereby improving an individual's self-esteem, and it is in the interest of the group as a whole to maintain this position. Groups compete to be different from each other in highly positive and creative ways, and this motivation for self-enhancement drives individuals to want to be members of highly-regarded groups, and also to have the opportunity for movement from a lower status group to one of higher status – the social mobility belief system – although this 'passing' from one group to another is only possible where intergroup boundaries are permeable (Hogg & Vaughan, 2005, p. 411). If this passing between groups is not possible, then the group can try to ensure that those attributes which define it are positive ones, or they can focus attention on other groups which are perceived as less prestigious so that in comparison they look better. Groups may also recognise that the entire basis on which their group is considered to be of lower status is neither rational nor fair, and this may encourage direct competition between groups.

Uncertainty reduction

The second motivation is that of uncertainty reduction. Individuals feel comfortable knowing how to react and behave in different social situations, and with an awareness of their social position. Uncertainty around this creates confusion and insecurity, so the drive to reduce ambiguity about the social world is high, and social categorisation is effective at limiting uncertainty as the individual can develop an understanding of group characteristics and prototype members. From this, accepted and approved behaviour can be predicted, giving the individual a pattern to follow if they wish for group acceptance. It appears that individuals who are most uncertain of themselves are more likely to want to belong to a distinctive group so as to give a clearer definition of themselves, with a 'sense of belonging'. Research has also shown that uncertainty reduction and self-enhancement directly influence each other. Individuals who are self-conceptually uncertain will identify equally with low or high status groups, whereas those who are highly self-conceptually certain are motivated to identify more with high status than low-status groups (Reid & Hogg, 2005). Another implication of this behaviour is that low status and subordinate groups do not seek to change their status and do not challenge higher status groups because to do so brings uncertainty and insecurity (Jost & Hunyadi, 2002).

Optimal Distinctiveness Theory

Brewer's 'Optimal Distinctiveness' theory (ODT) proposed that there was a third motive in social identity development. Brewer (1991) suggested that individuals have two opposing needs. The first is a need for inclusion, satisfied by being part of a group, whilst the second is for distinctiveness, satisfied by distinguishing oneself from others within a group. Individuals strike a balance between these two conflicting motives to achieve optimal distinctiveness.

Being a member of a smaller group over-satisfies the need for distinctiveness, so members struggle for greater inclusiveness. In large groups there is a heightened sense of inclusiveness so members want to be distinctive or 'special' within the group. From these findings, Brewer suggested that it is more satisfying to be a member of a medium-sized group rather than a very large or very small group.

Professional Identity

Professional identity is an extension of social identity, with the concept of professional identity referring to a set of values and attributes that differentiate one working role from another. These can be imposed either by those working within that role/group, or by outsiders (Sachs, 1999), so that professional identity provides a shared set of behaviours which enable the differentiation between professional groups. In the process of becoming a healthcare professional, students develop attitudes and values that align with those of the professional group they aspire to join. They explore the boundaries of how their profession is expected to behave and interact with other professional groups, and discover the limitations placed upon them by the concept of being a professional (Lingard, *et al.*, 2002).

There is much evidence to suggest that early clinical experience during the student years greatly influences professional identity development in healthcare, and that exposure not only encourages students to understand the roles and responsibilities of a range of healthcare professionals, but also to begin the process of identifying with a specific professional group. What is also thought to be important is the immersion in teams involving a range of different professionals rather than the chosen profession only, allowing the student to gain a different perspective of healthcare delivery (Helmich *et al.*, 2010).

Learning by observation is an underpinning concept of social learning theory; allowing the student to become part of a team, even in an observational capacity, allows them to witness team dynamics, individual responsibilities, and also how inter-personal conflict is managed. It is thought that this immersion has a profound affect on the way students perceive professional behaviour and develop their professional identity (Hafferty & Franks, 1994).

Construction of identity occurs via interaction with other professionals – the 'community of practice' – and participation in the team or group allows the student to develop group identity, bringing with it contextual comparisons with other groups in the working situation (Wenger, 1998). As the student becomes a member of the group, their position within the group is established, usually peripherally at first, but giving the student permission to participate in the group's work – a situation described by Lave and Wenger (1991) as 'legitimate peripheral participation'. This essentially means that the student is recognised as having a 'right' to be in the group but initially without a specified role, giving them the opportunity to observe individual roles within the wider context of the group.

Having gained this position within the group, the student must then become socialised, learning the patterns of behaviour, accepted modes of dress, and communication styles of the more experienced members. In healthcare, the group may consist of multiple disciplines or may be uni-disciplinary, but the differences and inter-actions between the professions are important in helping the student construct their perception of the relative status and value of each profession.

> The 'construction of the other' is an essential part of the professional categorisation process occurring at this point, and its importance cannot be overstated, for it is at this time that the student is laying down the foundation of their own professional identity in relation to themselves and to others, and once these impressions are formed, they are extremely difficult to alter (*Lingard et al., 2002*).

A further aspect of this professional socialisation is the encouragement to develop an understanding of what it is to be a professional. From this there is the recognition of self as being a representation of the profession, and this process is dependent on the existence of **role models**, which may be from the workplace, education, the home environment, or even the media. Clearly it is important that those who are role models provide a positive and constructive example as the perceptions and knowledge derived from them are central to the development of professional identity (Adams *et al.*, 2006). Interaction and reflection are also key aspects of this socialisation process, so discourse with other students and professionals will influence the developing identity. What is also important to remember is that this socialisation continues long after formal education finishes, so when moving into other work environments or joining other teams, professional identity can change in response to new challenges, problems, or situational change (Clark, 1997).

Interprofessional Relationships

One of the challenges of working within a group is the need to value the contribution of other group members, and this is particularly so in healthcare where multidisciplinary team working is predominant. In this case, the individual is not only aware of their own professional identity, but must also develop a framework of relative professional identities within which the individual can find their place. Social identity theory would suggest that being a member of a professional group means that the individual is categorised by their work, defining that individual in terms of their behaviours and attributes. In healthcare, this means that members of differing professions have a perception of the role, limits of practice, behaviours and even common characteristics of members from other professions, allowing issues such as stereotyping, prejudice, ethnocentrism, and favouritism to covertly become involved in working relationships.

Role conflict

Whilst generally it is recognised that multidisciplinary healthcare teams provide a rational and effective approach in service delivery (Cashman *et al.*, 2004), it has also long been accepted that there is conflict between the healthcare professions in relation to team roles (Watts *et al.*, 1990; Mizrahi & Abrahamson, 1985; Fox & Costle, 1994). Mariano (1989) stated:

It is naïve to bring highly diverse, skilled professionals together and assume, that by calling this group a team, it will act like a team.

Expanding on this notion, there is also discussion on whether physicians and non-medical clinicians are complementary or competitive in practice, this being reflected by either collaborative or parallel working practices (Grumbach & Coffman, 1998; Cashman *et al.*, 2004). It is clear that a multidisciplinary team is much more than a collection of highly trained professionals, and it is unwise to ignore the influence of social identity and group categorisation on both inter-professional and inter-personal relationships.

Three factors appear to hinder interdisciplinary relationships:

- goal and role conflict
- decision-making which does not involve all team members
- poor interpersonal communication.

Goal conflict arises where individuals hold different values, or disagree about how the value should be defined and interpreted. The conflict can become personal and emotional, making it difficult to resolve. These values may arise from personal, religious, or professional beliefs, so trust and respect is not endemic, value differences are not communicated, subverting team function. **Role conflict** includes misconceptions about the role of other professionals, role ambiguity, overlapping competencies and responsibilities, and stereotyping of other disciplines. Several factors have been identified that interfere with interdisciplinary working, such as poor inter-discipline communication, confusion over responsibility, ignorance of the conceptual basis of practice of another discipline, and a lack of trust and confidence in the ability and scope of other disciplines (Newberger, 1976).

A clear and realistic knowledge of one's own discipline is essential so that one can view how that discipline can contribute to the whole. When an individual feels 'safe' and secure from a professional viewpoint they are better positioned to act as an advocate for their profession, communicating strengths, limitations, and potential areas for contribution. However, the influence of separate, specialised and focused education can create professionals with the belief that their profession has the right to dominate other groups, and early socialisation within their own professional group can leave these individuals with significant feelings of superiority, which are then difficult to overcome. This separateness in education means that many professionals are unaware of the scope of practice, expertise, responsibilities, and competencies of other disciplines (Leathard, 2003). In an ideal situation students would be taught that no single professional group is predominant, and that overlapping of professional boundaries is acceptable without being confrontational and antagonistic.

A further issue in creating conflict is '**social proximity**'. Bruce (1980) suggested that differences in social status arising from historical factors and social distance created difficulties over co-operation between individuals from different professions. From the brief discussion above it can be clearly seen that the reduction of role conflict is essential for a team to function effectively. Ducanis and Golin (1979) suggested a number of steps which could be taken to overcome role conflict:

1. clarification of the expectations and perceptions of each other

2. identification of professional competencies

3. exploration of areas where responsibility over-laps

4. negotiation of role assignment.

This would allow the different professions to recognise and accept the value of each other's input, and highlight areas of practice where more than one profession may be able to contribute and collaborate. A further method of reducing role conflict is to approach professional education, with appropriate inter-professional learning being the foundation and starting point rather than a later addition. Learning together in formal pre-registration training, as well as in post-registration continual professional development allows the exploration of roles, shared knowledge, as well as identification of uniqueness.

Decision making

Effective decision making in teams requires a clear definition of the problem; clarity of member roles and their level of involvement in the decision; sufficient and relevant data about the problem; the availability of a range of options and alternatives; testing various options; and the commitment to carry out specified responsibilities. This is best achieved through respect for all members' contributions and expertise, constructive feedback, and shared responsibility for the outcome. This process does not always have to involve every team member with every decision, and neither is complete agreement from every team member essential, but each member must have an equal opportunity to influence the outcome. It is also important to be aware that leadership for decisions does not always need to rest with the same individual, and leadership can rotate depending on the situation.

Poor management of the decision-making process leads to decision error and decision obstruction (Mariano, 1989). This occurs because of a lack of clarity in identifying the problem, the roles of differing team members, and their relative involvement in the process. By not providing the opportunity for all team members to have input there is a danger that insufficient information is available and also that alternative options are not explored. Team members do not feel included in the process and can become frustrated at feeling powerless, lose interest, and make future decisions without consulting the rest of the team, leading to fragmentation and distrust.

Interpersonal communication

Improvement in inter-professional relationships relies on good communication. The freedom to share ideas without fear of ridicule, understanding aspirations, dealing constructively with disagreement and providing fair but clear feedback underpins this, which requires team members to value and respect each other. In an ideal team community individuals listen to each other, and negotiation rather than imposition prevails. Where one professional group, or even a single individual, acts autocratically, then power struggles will emerge and ultimately be destructive, with less assertive individuals being unable to express their opinions. However, effective communication also requires the team to regularly re-evaluate itself, but if the focus becomes purely about the process of team working, then the original goal of the team is lost. Healthcare teams that do not communicate effectively may still consist of dedicated and motivated members, but they fail to work together in the best interests of their patients and lose sight of the team's goals, a situation highlighted by the Kennedy Report (2001) from the Bristol Royal Infirmary Public Inquiry.

Summary

As has been mentioned previously, the development of a professional identity is closely related to how an individual develops their social identity, the professional identity being one of many which are potentially salient. Social Identity Theory would suggest that this creates difficulties in healthcare where different professional groups will compete for dominance and exhibit classical 'in-group' and 'out-group' characteristics so that group members can feel positive about themselves, and create a 'safe' environment. The need for self-enhancement and positive distinctiveness creates competition between professionals, and because it is unusual in healthcare for an individual to move from one professional group to another, professional groups who perceive themselves to be of higher status will try and dominate less prestigious groups. These comparisons are frequently based on a poor understanding of another professional group, creating conflict and distrust. To try and overcome these barriers it would seem sensible to prevent formation of absolute group distinctions and mis-perceptions, which requires examination of the educational processes employed in healthcare training. Early socialisation between different professional groups, with shared learning environments and encouragement of collaborative working, is already fairly widespread in UK Higher Education Institutions, but it remains to be seen whether this is effective in the long term in reducing inter-disciplinary dissonance and encouraging truly collaborative and effective team work in healthcare.

References

Adams, K., Hean, S., Sturgis, P. and Clark, J. (2006). 'Investigating the factors influencing professional identity of first-year health and social care students' in *Learning in Health and Social Care*: **5**(2) 55–68.

Allport, G.W. (1979). *The Nature of Prejudice: 25th Anniversary.* New York, USA: Basic Books.

Brewer, M.B. (1991). 'The social self: on being the same and different at the same time' in *Personality and Social Psychology Bulletin,* **17**(5): 475–482.

Brewer, M.B. (2003). *Intergroup Relations* 2nd ed. Buckingham: Open University Press.

Brown, R. (2000). 'Social Identity Theory: past achievements, current problems and future challenges' in *European Journal of Social Psychology*, **30**: 745–778.

Bruce, N. (1980). *Teamwork for Preventative Care.* Chichester: Wiley & Sons.

Bruner, J.S. (1957). 'On perceptual readiness' in *Psychological Review* **64**(2): 123–151.

Cashman, S.B., Reidy, P., Cody, K. and Lemay, C.A. (2004). 'Developing and measuring progress toward collaborative, integrated, interdisciplinary healthcare teams' in *Journal of Interprofessional Care*. **18** (2): 183–196.

Clark, P. (1997). 'Values in healthcare professional socialisation: implications for geriatric education in interdisciplinary teamwork' in *The Gerontologist*, **37**(4): 441–451.

Ducanis, A.J. and Golin, A.K. (1979). *The Interdisciplinary Healthcare Team: A Handbook.* Germantown, USA: Aspen Systems Corporation.

Fox, R.D. and Costle, K.A. (1994). *Health professionals' expectations of physicians. Report of the survey of selected professionals in Ontario.* EFPO Working Paper.

Grumbach, K. and Coffman, J. (1998). 'Physicians and nonphysician clinicians: complements or competitors?'

in *Journal of the American Medical Association*, **280**(9): 825–826.

Hafferty, F.W. and Franks, R. (1994). 'The hidden curriculum, ethics teaching, and the structure of medical education' in *Academic Medicine*, **69**(11): 861–871.

Helmich, E., Derksen, E., Prevoo, M., Laan, R., Bolhuis, S. and Koopmans, R. (2010). 'Medical students professional identity development in an early nursing attachment' in *Medical Education*, **44**(7): 674–682.

Hewstone, M., Rubin, M. and Willis, H. (2002). 'Intergroup bias' in *Annual Review of Psychology*. **53**(1): 575–604.

Hogg, M.A. (2006). 'Social Identity Theory' in *Contemporary Social Psychological Theories*, ed. P.J. Burkep. 111. California: Stanford University Press.

Hogg, M.A. and Vaughan, G.M. (2005). *Social Psychology* 4th ed. London: Pearson Education Ltd.

Hopkins, N. and Moore, C.(2001). 'Categorizing the neighbours: Identity, distance, and stereotyping' in *Social Psychology Quarterly*, **64**(3): 239–52.

Jost, J.T. and Hunyadi, O. (2002). 'The psychology of system justification and the palliative function of ideology' in *European Review of Social Psychology*, **13**: 111–153.

Kennedy, I. (2001). *The Report of the Public Enquiry into Children's Heart Surgery at the Bristol Royal Infirmary, 1984-1995 Learning from Bristol*. London: The Stationery Office.

Lave, J. and Wenger, E. (1991). *Situated Learning: Legitimate peripheral participation*. Cambridge: Cambridge University Press.

Leathard, A. (2003). *Interprofessional Collaboration: From Policy to Practice in Health and Social Care*. Hove, East Sussex: Brunner-Routledge.

Lickel, B., Hamilton, D L , Wieczorkowska, G., Lewis, A., Sherman, S.J. and Uhles, A.N. (2000). Varieties of groups and the perception of group entitativity, *Journal of Personality and Social Psychology*, **78**(2): 223–246.

Lingard, L., Reznick, R., DeVito, I. and Espin, S. (2002). 'Forming professional identities on the healthcare team: discursive construction of the "other" in the operating room' in *Medical Education*. **36**(8): 728–734.

Mackie, D.M. and Smith, E.R. (1998). 'Intergroup relations: Insights from a theoretically integrative approach' in *Psychological Review*, **105**(3): 499–529.

Mariano, C. (1989). 'The case for interdisciplinary collaboration' in *Nursing Outlook*, Nov/Dec: 286–289.

Mizrahi, T. and Abrahamson, J. (1985). 'Sources of strain between physicians and social workers: Implications for social workers in healthcare settings' in *Social Work in Healthcare*, **10**(3) 33–51.

Newberger, E.A. (1976). 'A physician's perspective on the interdisciplinary management of child abuse' in *Pyschiatric Opinion*, **2**: 13–18.

Oakes, P.J., Turner, J.C. and Haslam, S.A. (1991). 'Perceiving people as group members: The role of fit in the salience of social categorizations' in *British Journal of Social Psychology*, **30**(2):, pp. 125–144.

Reid, S.A. and Hogg, M.A. (2005). 'Uncertainty reduction, self-enhancement, and in-group identification' in *Personality and Social Psychology Bulletin*, **31**: 1–14.

Sachs, J. (1999). Teacher Professional Identity: Competing discourses, competing outcomes. Conference presentation. Australian Association of Research in Education (AARE) Conference, Melbourne, November 1999.

Salzarulo, L. (2004). Formalizing self-categorization theory to simulate the formation of social groups. Conference Paper. The Second European Social Simulation Association Conference, 16–19th September, Valladolid, Spain.

Savage, M. (2002). 'Social exclusion and class analysis' in *Social Differences and Divisions*, eds. P. Braham and L. James, p.62. Oxford: Blackwell Publishers.

Tajfel, H. and Turner, J. (1979). 'An integrative theory of intergroup conflict' in *The Social Psychology of Intergroup Relations* (1996), eds. W.G. Austin and S. Worchel, pp. 33–47. Monterey, California: Brooks/Cole.

Tajfel, H. and Turner, J.C. (1986). 'The social identity theory of intergroup behaviour' in *Psychology of Intergroup Relations*, eds. S. Worchel and W.G. Austin, pp. 7–24. Chicago: Nelson-Hall.

Turner, J.C. (1996). 'Self-categorization Theory' in *The Blackwell Encyclopedia of Social Psychology*, eds. A.S.R. Manstead and M. Hewstone. Blackwell Reference Online <http://www.blackwellreference.com/public/book?id=g9780631202899_g978063120289921 (accessed 31/05/12).

Voci, A. (2006). 'Relevance of social categories, depersonalisation, and group processes: Two field tests of self-categorisation theory' in *European Journal of Social Psychology*, **36**(1): 73–90.

Watts, D.T., McCaulley, B.L. and Priefer, B.A. (1990). 'Physician-nurse conflict: lessons from a clinical experience' in *Journal of the American Geriatric Society*, **38**(10): 1151–1152.

Wenger, E. (1998). *Communities of Practice. Learning, Meaning and Identity*. Cambridge: Cambridge University Press.

Chapter Two
Clinical Professional Practice

Shelagh Keogh

"Would you tell me please, which way I ought to go from here?"
"That depends on where you want to get to," said the Cat
"I don't much care where —" said Alice
"Then it doesn't matter which way you go," said the Cat
"— so long as I get somewhere," Alice added as an explanation.
"Oh, you are sure to do that," said the Cat "if you only walk long enough."

Lewis Carroll, *Alice's Adventures in Wonderland* (1865)

Defining Professionalism

Most people would agree that professionalism is a philosophy or a notional standard by which a person can be judged or can aspire to be perceived in their approach and behaviour in the context of clinical professional practice. Far from being a tangible, concrete object which one can see, hear or touch, it is a philosophically socially constructed ideal. The foundations of this underpinning philosophy were constituted by the dominant professions of law and medicine. A simple operational definition is that professionalism is the behaviour of a professional within a profession, a profession being an occupation that requires a high level of skill and understanding, usually necessitating formal qualifications from an accrediting body and also the regulatory body Codes of Practice. In this sense any transgression from those standards would mean a member was by definition unprofessional or not behaving in a professional manner.

Conceptual Models of Professionalism

There are many conceptual models that have been developed to understand the phenomenon of professionalism. As far back as 1915, Abraham Flexner outlined criteria for defining a profession and produced a seminal work, 'Is Social Work a Profession?'. This work has been developed over the last century.

> *"Professions involve essentially intellectual operations with large individual responsibility; they derive their raw material from science and learning; this material they work up to a practical and definitive end; they possess an educationally communicable technique; they tend to self-organization; they are becoming increasingly altruistic in motivation."* (Flexner, 1915, p. 10)

The foundations of this fundamentally original thinking were greatly influenced by the dominant professions of law and medicine at the time. When Flexner was constructing his paper on professional behaviour he was considering various disciplines, social work at the time did not have professional status but had developed significantly as a subject area. Podiatric medicine's history is also significant when we consider the only relatively recent closure of the profession in terms of the need for professional registration.

Greenwood (1957) refined Flexner's work into five attributes of a profession: systematic theory; authority; community sanction; ethical codes; a culture.

The following aspects of these two conceptual models, in relation to the development of the practice of podiatry, will be discussed below:

- body of knowledge
- community sanction
- professional cohesion or organisation
- professional culture
- institutionalised altruism.

Body of Knowledge

Defining professionalism with an emphasis on scientific knowledge could be interpreted as implying that the professional should be working from one body of knowledge. Very few knowledge sources of professional disciplines focus on one body of knowledge; medicine, in particular, understands that many knowledge bases affect a client's presentation of illness, for example economics, political developments, psychology, and social structures.

In 1915 the university sector represented a very different infrastructure from our current institutional system and some professional disciplines were not considered essential enough to be given departmental status. The clinical practice of podiatry was one such discipline and the emergence of the profession in terms of knowledge and contribution to health and medicine over the last century has played a key role in the recognition of podiatric medicine as a professional discipline. The notion of accessible healthcare and the acknowledgement that the discipline of podiatric medicine could play a major role in the prevention of lower limb morbidity and pathology have paved the way for the further development of professional identity.

Community Sanction

Within medicine, in particular, doctors' professional bodies do have a public sanction to administer and govern professional practice, and other professional disciplines, such as nursing, have followed this trajectory. The behaviour and practice of these professionals have also been required to comply with the standards of regulatory bodies in order to frame and guide their approach. Nursing and the medical profession maintain their standards by ensuring the ability to practice is only given to those with membership of their professional body who have demonstrated competence and continuous professional development. Any organisation having the ability to determine the criteria for membership to a profession is also fundamentally responsible for the implementation of ethical practice in relation to equality and human rights.

The appropriate level of competency is usually a prerequisite for the admission to a professional body and podiatric medicine is no exception. In theory, indirect discrimination can exist in the form of cultural ignorance of its participants. So for example the ability to achieve the level of competence may also necessitate the achievements of verbal entrance examinations in relation to basic communication skills fit for clinical practice. Bias could manifest in relation to certain accents or cultural representations, and the fiscal cost in achieving the prerequisite level of competence could be such that it discriminates against some levels of our social structures.

Having sole rights over technical issues may also result in a dominant group using their religious or cultural norms as a measure for decision making. For example, if within a professional discipline a high level of practitioner cohesiveness is achieved, the fundamental danger is that narrowness of approach and bias in thinking is a net result of '**Groupthink**'.

Groupthink Theory

Irving (1971) carried out research into 'Groupthink Theory'. The main principle behind the theory is that the more consensual agreement and the greater the degree of belief between members of a policy-making in-group, the greater the danger that independent critical thinking will be replaced by groupthink, which is likely to result in irrational and dehumanising actions against out-groups.

Professional Cohesion or Organisation

Specific organisations such as the National Health Service are required to employ clinical professions for whom registration with a professional body is a prerequisite for being able to practice within their clinical discipline. Podiatric practitioners in the United Kingdom are expected to have a qualification recognised by the Society of Chiropodists and Podiatrists and also be registered with the Health Professions Council. This ensures accountability within a professional framework which is epitomised by strong cohesion between its members. Membership of the vast majority of professional regulatory bodies ensures access to participation in activities such as conferences, branch organisation meetings, sharing of best practice and the dissemination of new and emerging practices within specific clinical fields of practice.

Within the context of podiatric medicine in the United Kingdom a rigorous process of accreditation and regulation surrounds the award of all programmes of study, regardless of whether they are developed for delivery at undergraduate level, postgraduate level or specifically for the context of continuing professional development. By placing the body at the centre of professional regulation this also secures the ability of the Society of Chiropodists and Podiatrists to deal quickly and efficiently in addressing any fitness to practice issues raised via the Health Professions Council.

Professional culture

The development of a language and discourse which effectively ensure the communication of concepts, theory and practice can serve to provide professional boundaries which are often deemed inaccessible by those outside the profession. Often this discourse develops in a manner which can be directly correlated with the deepening complexity of knowledge underpinning a professional discipline such as podiatric medicine.

Institutionalised altruism

Podiatric medicine is a discipline which can claim that members of the profession clearly engage in their professional activities not purely to earn a living but also to make a valuable contribution to society on a bigger scale, the concept of which is being popularised and advocated within recent policy.

Many authors have examined the various motivations for altruistic involvement within the volunteer sector. Hackl *et al.* (2007) researched this area of professional practice and concluded that there are no unambiguous definitions of altruistic work. The kind of benefit expected by individuals engaging in such activity can be grouped under an investment model encompassing three core areas, namely:

- the ability to contribute to the lives of others, which can be definitively framed as self worth (Meier, 2006)
- a perceived enjoyment of working in terms of personal satisfaction, the notion of increased self-determination and the contribution which work makes to the feeling of competence (Argyle, 1999); Deci, 1975; Frey 1997; Deci and Ryan 2000)
- the feeling of having done something 'good' (Andrewoni, 1990)

The volunteering act can be argued as creating an opportunity to benefit as an individual. Although Abraham Flexner's seminal work was first published in 1915 one can still clearly identify the sentiments and values in all professional codes of conduct regardless of professional distinction. At this point, it is also useful to consider private practice within clinical professional practice for podiatrists, and the debate that altruistic elements of practice can contribute directly to the role of the podiatrists in their wider contribution to society as a whole.

Codes of Conduct

The vast majority of professional bodies regulate membership by the compulsory sponsorship of a code of conduct. The code is a standard which guides and regulates the behaviour of the members and within the context of healthcare usually governs issues surrounding 'Fitness to Practice'. Any member of the Society of Chiropodists and Podiatrists not adhering to a professional code of conduct in terms of fitness to practice is required to account for their practice and can potentially be asked to leave or indeed be required to leave the professional body. This has legalistic ramifications in terms of the consequences of the actions of podiatric practitioners. Since the practice of podiatric medicine is now restricted to those members of the profession registered with the Society of Chiropodists and Podiatrists, the consequences of this to the future professional practice of individuals can be devastating. It is here that the clear differentiation between protocols and guidelines should be managed in dealing with individual patients and their presenting podiatric conditions.

The perception of professional disciplines, including podiatric medicine, hinges upon the agenda drivers taken from different stakeholder viewpoints. These viewpoints will be based on stakeholder needs including economic concerns. Hence the effect of the professional status of podiatry on the fiscal viability of care provision will be significant.

Defining and Framing Stakeholders

With regards to the patient base, in terms of a profession such as podiatric medicine, the patient can be both the recipient of the treatment or the purchaser of the treatment (the central government or the individual tax payer).

Within the context of podiatric medicine, the patient's main drivers are:
- Whether need can be addressed with an acceptable level of quality within the context in which it is being offered. This situational context can differ significantly on a societal level, on an international basis.

- Whether the cost will be such that the service or goods supplied are considered affordable and economically viable.

The podiatric practitioner's primary drivers are:

- Whether continuing professional development courses are sufficient in theoretical knowledge transferability to be applied at the front line of patient care. (This theme is further developed in the chapter on strategic curriculum design for podiatric medicine, Chapter 6.)

The podiatric educational provider's drivers are:

- Whether there is evidence from stakeholders and practitioners to inform the curriculum content of programmes of study in podiatric medicine.
- Whether educational packages can be truly regarded as being strategic and needs-led in order to meet the specific needs of practitioners working at the front line of patient care.

The prosecutors of the law's drivers are:

- Whether the laws implemented are sufficient to protect those members of the public who depend on the practice of podiatric clinicians, educators and researchers.
- Whether those laws implemented are sufficiently supported with rigorous reporting and accountability procedures to be able to support those affected by acts which are socially and professionally unacceptable.

The Society of Chiropodists and Podiatrists (i.e. the professional body's) drivers are:

- Whether podiatric practice protects the rights of all stakeholders.
- Whether the facilitation of the protection and enhancement of the knowledge base underpinning the practice of podiatric medicine is centrally enabled.

Codes of conduct are professional standards and as such should be in a dynamic state of constant re-evaluation in order to establish processes of critical reflexivity on professional practice, the incorporation of best practice procedures and address of any ethical dilemmas arising. The starting point for a code of conduct should be at a point in professional history when there is sufficient knowledge from a breadth of practice to capture good professional approaches and strategies.

In devising specific codes of conduct, many organisations produce highly philosophical, symbolic and ceremonial devices which are essentially unsuitable for implementation in practice. This ambiguous and ill conceived process of developing codes can create significantly more issues than are typically resolved, particularly when codes exist in direct contradiction or competition with one another. A typical example of this is the development of a code which declares that all professional members must ensure they work towards the needs of the clients, alongside another code which declares that all professional members must ensure they work towards the needs of the professional body. It cannot necessarily be assumed that both the professional body and the client have mutually compatible desires and needs. These conflicts of interest should be resolved prior to any implementation at the front line of patient care provision. Again this is where the clear distinction between protocols and guidelines is necessary in terms of allowing ethical and legal practice which permits podiatric practitioners the flexibility to individualise care pathways.

The rationale for the development and implementation of codes is primarily the prevention of problems. This does not essentially prevent problems but the adoption of specific codes within the context of podiatric practice will contribute to the process of overcoming issues in practice. What is notable here is that one code may not be effective or even possible for implementation across all nationalities and cultures. Cultural norms and values can affect the adoption of principles built into a code of conduct. A typical example of this is the Hippocratic Oath. At one time in its existence the oath adopted the principle that a doctor could aid a patient to commit suicide but they could not facilitate a patient to execute an abortion; today in the UK the governmental and societal stance has effectively been reversed.

The adoption of a code of conduct by a professional body cannot lead to the assumption that the profession is working as required by the specific code implemented. The implementation of any code requires also a mechanism to ensure the conduct of personnel is at the prerequisite professional standards. Ensuring a professional body deals with its non-compliant members is difficult in execution, especially in professions where nepotism is an issue. When professionals work together the desired bond of the profession can have positive and negative outcomes; one of the negatives is that the unacceptable performance of members would need to be highlighted to the appropriate committee or regulatory board. Even personal relationships may impact upon professional groups and their identities. Many professionals marry people from within their own profession and subsequently their children become professionals within the same discipline so in a relatively short space of time people know others or become the friends of people who know others and so on. The emotional and ethical dilemma of being aware of a friend or colleague performing at a suboptimal level is at best difficult and at worst impossible to address.

Ethical Dilemmas

One key responsibility of a professional regulatory body is to take a lead in addressing ethically sensitive issues and situations arising. An ethical situation can be defined as one in which the practitioner has to make a decision involving judgements of value or rights. The potential impact of such decisions upon stakeholders is an enormous responsibility. It is impossible to predict and address every such situation in advance, especially given continuing changes in technology and ways of working, which can give rise to unanticipated consequences. The need for accountability can therefore affect the rates of innovation and change in the profession.

In this respect professional bodies can act as a central hub for advice in the facilitation of decision making in ethical dilemmas. As professionals, podiatric practitioners cannot avoid ethical dilemmas since they are an integral part of healthcare provision; indeed some ethical dilemmas may have personal consequences. Restrictions in patient confidentiality, data protection laws and the notion of informed consent all impact upon the ability to practice freely and all necessitate the consideration of the parameters of practice within which clinicians may operate.

Emerging Technology and Expertise

Many professionals depend on the use of technology. Within the practice of podiatric medicine the last twenty-five years have seen the emergence of an array of treatment modalities and assessment mechanisms which have revolutionised the profession as a whole. The field of podiatric biomechanics is perhaps the greatest example of such innovation and the profession has undertaken seminal work in the field of human gait analysis and ambulation, which now serves as a means of informing patient management pathways in a manner once only imaginable. There are however, drawbacks to the implementation of technology within clinical professional practice. Skill development depends on podiatric practitioners who have specific psychomotor and cognitive awareness of technological processes in relation to the medical need of patients and developing competence in the use of new and emerging technology is an issue. The notion of systems failure has also impacted significantly on the potential for human error since technology is ultimately dependent upon the competence of its operators.

'Systems failure'

In 1990, Reason described two theories of failure which were categorised as active and latent failure.

- **Active Failure** is the direct result of those individual actions which can be directly attributed to the cause of the failure – for example a podiatrist who transfers infection from one toe to another through a lack of regard for recognised sterilisation procedures (Reason, 1990).

- **Latent Failure** differs significantly in that it is error in process or infrastructures which are not discovered until the window of opportunity arises for a related set of circumstances to coincide. For example, it could be that operating policies are ambiguous, user testing ineffective or more commonly poor communication might limit understanding of the prerequisites for correct usage of newly implemented technology. Latent errors are thus much more difficult to detect, prevent and ultimately comprehend.

Bennett *et al.* (2002) raised key issues of failure from a stakeholder perspective, effectively categorising three main stakeholders in the process:

- **User Perspective** – this is essentially where the product fails because it is difficult to use and it is not fit for purpose (which essentially mirrors Reason's classification of Active Failure).

- **Client Perspective** – this is where a product fails if the production cost is too great, where trust in the product is eroded or it effectively does not deliver what was expected to a consumer seeking an appropriate product.

- **Developer Perspective** – this is where the product is not well enough developed to address the specific needs of the consumer or more commonly if practitioners use equipment for a purpose other than that for which it was specifically designed.

There are several considerations worthy of note here, initially that it is the professional responsibility of the practitioner upon accepting the need to use equipment to ensure they are competent in its use and to give feedback to suppliers as necessary.

Opportunities to Improve Professional Practice

Reflective practice and more significantly the ability to be critically reflexive is the characteristic which epitomises the ultimate professional, regardless of their professional discipline. This is an issue further discussed in Chapter 7, but which also is clearly identifiable within any discussion of clinical professional practice. The majority of employees are afforded the opportunity to take part in an individual process of appraisal on an annual basis. Institutional culture is significant in this instance where the notion of being free from negative judgement on practice can be significant in how comfortable the majority of practitioners are in the process of reflection. Ownership of professional development thus becomes a significant issue which will be discussed at length in subsequent chapters.

Basic Personal Reflection and Ownership of Continuing Professional Development

Being straightforward in approach and embracing a core ability to demonstrate self awareness is essentially the hallmark of productive reflective practice. One straightforward mechanism of personal reflection is to produce a basic framework of questions with which to structure engagement with the process. For example on a daily or weekly basis it might be as simple as:

- Which tasks have been undertaken/which clinical procedures have been performed today?
- How can the quality of the outcome from these tasks best be described?
- Did the execution of the tasks incorporate up-to-date good practice?
- If there is a need to repeat any of the processes or procedures, is there a demonstrable need to change practice?
- Is there a recognisable need to improve the skill base currently adopted in practice?

In comparison an annual evaluation might be extended to frame practice provision with such key questions as:

- What has been achieved well this year?
- What could been improved in performance this year?
- What sort of vocational or professional development has been completed this year?
- Is there evidence of the active incorporation of learning from vocational training into practice this year?
- Which training needs can be established for the forthcoming year?
- Which objectives can be set for the forthcoming year which will best fit the training needs identified?

In situations requiring a degree of self awareness, such as in personal development planning, identifying complex and intellectually based issues may not be as effective as identifying straightforward and simple aspects of practice which can be readily addressed to change and improve practice. For example, a straightforward reflection on our ability to engage and interact with patients can make a significant difference to the mechanisms with which we engage clinically with patients from a diverse array of backgrounds in an equally diverse array of clinical contexts and settings. It is often the process of being institutionalised by engaging daily in task driven exercises and target driven agendas which may prevent practitioners from engaging in basic processes of self reflection.

Linking to the Concept of Professional Identity

In the previous chapter on professional identity, several theories have been presented to explain how professions are perceived and how professionalism is demonstrated by the individual practitioner. The stereotyping which surrounds professional communities is an integral part of their perception by wider society and indeed can be a source of professional identity. In terms of clinical professional practice, there are various mechanisms by which podiatric medicine might be perceived as a profession. Personal appearance is one practical aspect of professional identity which can create both positive and negative perceptions of the podiatric practitioner in relation to their overall credibility as a healthcare professional.

Professionalism entails giving the impression of respect and dignity in all daily interactions. It should be remembered that it is not only verbal communication which is indicative of the ability to be professional. Body language can also dictate much of how we are perceived and including facial expressions and overall personal demeanour. Cultural and social skills are equally important at the front line of patient care in clinical professional practice in podiatric medicine. Having a basic understanding and appreciation of the need to be respectful for another's culture is an easy and manageable mechanism of building social cohesion. In terms of the fundamentals of communication skills, miscommunication is all too easy and as already outlined, it is not only verbally that we communicate. Observing the impact of our interaction with others can be a significant lesson in understanding how our clinical professional practice is appropriate to the level of healthcare provision with which we engage. The differentiation between knowledge and wisdom is also significant at this stage, with the recognition of the need to travel on a continuous journey of self-improvement a pivotal part of the latter.

Conclusion

The conscientious podiatric practitioner is always ready to reflect and to improve on current practice in the light of new and innovative approaches to professional practice. This alongside a willingness to share new approaches and to contribute to the development of others by sharing best practice is one mechanism by which this can be achieved. The following chapter on Mentorship for Podiatric Practice expands this theme in a significantly greater level of detail.

References

Andreoni, J. (1990). 'Impure altruism and donations to public goods: A theory of warm-glow giving' in *Economic Journal*, **100**(401): 464–477.

Argyle, M. (1999). 'Causes and correlates of happiness', in *Well-Being: The Foundations of Hedonic Psychology,* eds. D. Kahneman, E. Diener and N. Schwarz. New York: RussellSage Foundation.

Bennett, S., McRobb, S. and Farmer, R. (2002). *Object-oriented Systems Analysis and Design using UML*, 2nd edition. Maidenhead: McGraw-Hill.

Buchanan, D. and Huczynski, A. (1997). *Organisational Behaviour: An Introductory Text*, 3rd edition. Hemel Hempstead: Prentice Hall.

Deci, E. L. (1975). *Intrinsic Motivation*. New York: Plenum Press.

Deci, E.L. and Ryan, R.M. (2000). 'The "what" and "why" of goal pursuits: Human needs and the self-determination of behavior' in *Psychological Inquiry,* **11**(4): 227–268.

Flexner, A. (1915) 'Is Social Work a Profession?' An address to the National Conference of Charities and Corrections, Baltimore.
Available at: archive.org/stream/CU31924014006617#page/n1/mode/2up (Accessed 04/07/12)

Frey, B.S. (1997). 'A constitution for knaves crowds out civic virtues' in *Economic Journal,* **107**(443): 1043–1053.

Greenwood, E. (1957). 'Attributes of a profession' in *Social Work* **2**(3): 45–55.

Hackl, F., Halla, M. and Pruckner, G.J. (2007). *Volunteering and Income – The Fallacy of the Good Samaritan*? Kyklos, Wiley-Blackwell.

Irving, J. (1971). 'Groupthink' in *Psychology Today,* **11**(1): 43–46.

Meier, S. (2006). *The Economics of Non-selfish Behaviour: Decisions to Contribute Money to Public Goods,* Cheltenham: Edward Elgar Publishing.

Reason, J.T. (1990). *Human Error.* Cambridge: Cambridge University Press.

Reason, J.T. (2000). 'Human error: models and management' in *British Medical Journal,* **320**(7237): 768–70.

Chapter Three
Mentorship in Podiatric Practice

Dr John Fulton

Contextualising Mentorship

In many ways the term mentorship has become something of a buzzword and is one which arises in a number of settings. The expression 'mentor' was first used in Homer's 'Odyssey': Mentor was a friend of Odysseus, who placed his son in the charge of Mentor when he went off to fight in the Trojan wars (Andrews & Wallis, 1999).

In professional healthcare, the term mentorship is used to describe a relationship more akin to the concept of practice supervision which involves monitoring the development of the student in the clinical setting. In the business world the term is used, in a different sense, to describe the relationship of a junior person with a more senior colleague who will guide and advise them often throughout the early part of their career. Contact may not be ideal in terms of the specific dedication of time to the process but the mentor is usually around to guide and support them for a suitable and mutually agreeable length of time. Another increasingly popular aspect of mentorship in practice is that in which people in disadvantaged areas take on the role of mentoring a young person and subsequently become a surrogate sibling in terms of their relationship to the person they mentor. Various approaches can be termed mentorship but the definitive use of the term remains debatable.

In the 1980s, nursing and midwifery took up the term to describe the supervisory relationship of the (pre-registration) student and their clinical supervisor (Andrews & Wallis, 1999). Whilst in the other health professions this term is not used with quite the same definitive precision as in nursing and midwifery it will be used throughout this chapter as a straightforward means of operationally defining the concept and process. The aim of this is, very specifically, to describe the relationship between a student and the practitioner who will assist and guide the student in the clinical setting. This is not to say that a podiatrist may not develop a long-term mentorship relationship with a more senior colleague as part of their on-going professional development. However, the student in practice will raise many different issues and it is this aspect which will be the focus of this chapter.

Roles of the Mentor

Harden and Crosby (2000) in discussing medical education discuss the role of the teacher and outline six key areas that see the teacher as:

- an information provider
- a role model
- a facilitator
- an assessor
- a planner (of the curriculum)
- a resource developer.

Whilst there are some significant differences between a lecturer in an academic post and the mentor, these roles are a helpful way of encapsulating the requirements of mentorship and it is a useful start to consider each one.

The mentor as an **information giver** needs to provide basic information to the student both about the practicalities of the clinical placement and the expectation anticipated from the student. There is a danger that the mentor will become so embedded in this role that they see themselves as the source of all information and it is important that the other roles gain some consideration.

The mentor also needs to be a **role model** especially within the discipline of podiatric medicine and the student can learn much from observing a suitably experienced practitioner, particularly around ways of dealing with a diverse array of situations, which commonly present in clinical practice. Part of this particular mentorship role lies in discussion and reflection upon how certain situations are handled and the direct translation of theory to practice.

People fundamentally learn by doing and the mentor needs to focus on the facilitation aspect of the role and ensure that the student is navigated towards gaining relevant information both in terms of finding out facts and being able to visit other people and departments. This element of the mentoring relationship gives fundamental responsibility for learning to the student with the mentor facilitating rather than dictating the process.

As an **assessor**, it is important that the mentor can use their skills to make a considered judgement about the students in terms of their strengths in skill development and those areas in which they may need to improve. Feedback is always important, the student requires regular feedback, but the course tutors also require feedback about the curriculum and its feasibility in practice.

Effective mentorship does not occur by chance and time needs to be spent in **logistical planning** for the student.

An integral part of planning lies in the **development of resources** which can be utilised by the student in the practice setting. With the development of internet resources this is a much less onerous task than it has been historically with several organisations willing to share best practice with a firm evidence base.

Whilst it is important to consider aspects of the mentor's role and it provides much insight as to what takes place in practice, it is perhaps also useful to consider some of the theoretical concepts which underpin the practice of mentorship, notably:

- Constructionist approaches to learning (Vygotsky, 1978)
- Emotional labour (Hochschild, 1983)
- Communities of practice (Lave and Wenger, 1991)
- Formative assessment (Black & Wiliam, 1998).

Constructionist Approaches to Learning

Traditionally, the teacher is seen as the fount of knowledge and as such is the person who imparts his or her knowledge to receptive students. In this sense the students are perceived as symbolic empty vessels waiting to be filled with knowledge and information. The teacher/mentor as an information provider is how many overseas students see the mentor's role as they often originate from a culture where the teacher is regarded as the holder of knowledge and as such must never be challenged in terms of their academic ability. This notion is far removed from the concept of mentorship. An oft quoted definition of mentor is that of Megginson and Clutterbuck (1995, p.13) who state that mentoring is:

> *off line help by one person to another in making significant transitions in knowledge, work or thinking.*

This definition goes further than merely imparting knowledge to the student and it implies a much wider approach to mentorship and placing emphasis on the theory to practice relationship and the application of acquired knowledge to the practice setting. Following this line of thinking a useful way of exploring the mentorship role is in terms of what education means for the individual.

Constructionist approaches see the learner not as a passive recipient into whom knowledge is poured but as someone who actively constructs and is motivated to develop their own working knowledge base.

Mezirow (1991), in his theory of transformative learning, discusses how through reflection on experience and discussion, the learner can challenge their traditional ways of thinking, change their perspectives and progressively move into new ways of learning and engagement with applying theory to practice. The mentor is key to this role as it is through discussion and facilitation characteristic of the formalised mentoring relationship that this (what Mezirow calls) transformative learning takes place.

The theory–practice gap

The 'Zone of Proximal Development' (Vygotsky, 1978) is a concept used to describe the space between what students actually know and what they are required to know or in terms of skill development between what they can safely practice now and what they are required to do but cannot do independently. The metaphor of structural 'scaffolding' is used to describe the support, which is provided for students and then strategically and gradually withdrawn until the learner can practice the particular skill independently. It is also a useful way of bridging the theory–practice gap (Spouse, 2001) by providing support allowing the individual to explore what works and what does not work in practice and the translation of their theoretical ideas and understanding to the practice of podiatric medicine.

'Advanced organisers'

Another theoretical idea is that of 'Advanced Organisers' this comes from the work of David Ausubel (1963) who emphasised the importance of finding out what the learners know and what they think it is useful to learn. To use a cliché, people 'don't know what they don't know' and in practice it is a strategic process of negotiation where the mentor finds out what the learner presently knows and needs or is motivated to learn, subsequently working with him or her to determine a formalised and achievable plan of action. The challenge for the mentor lies in the strategic management of the situation, as individuals must meet the requirements of their programme of study. It is not to say the learner is given total freedom to do whatever they want, rather they are equipped with the motivation to learn and consolidate and build upon pre-existing knowledge. In practice, however, students know what they need to learn and are required to do as part of a placement and are happy to fulfil what is expected of them. This approach allows them to determine and to some extent individualise their particular way of doing so.

Constructionist approaches also mean the learner can and should research and develop the knowledge base around subject areas and a significant role of the mentor is to act as a facilitator, who will direct and navigate the student in the direction of resource materials rather than give them this information directly. Clearly, on the level of social need, there are some things the mentor should tell the student such as where the refectory is or where they can get coffee. On a more serious note there are formalised protocols surrounding Health and Safety, which the student needs to know, and which must be imparted. The central message here is that the more self directed and active the student is in their engagement with the curriculum, the more they will actually learn and be able to apply theory to practice.

Phases in the mentorship relationship

One can deduce that the mentor–student relationship is a reciprocal one, which needs to be worked at on the part of both mentor and students. Cahill (1996)and Ali and Panther (2008) suggest that there are essentially three phases in the mentorship relationship, namely the **Initiation Phase**, the **Working Phase** and the **Termination Phase**.

The Initiation Phase is where the mentor and student are introduced to one another socially and professionally, where both the boundaries and the goals that the student wishes to achieve during the placement are set. It is the period of the 'advanced organiser' whereby the mentor finds out precisely what the student knows and how they will build on that pre-existing knowledge and develop the necessary skills and strategies relevant to their period of study.

The working phase is where the mentor provides the necessary metaphorical scaffolding which supports the students in their skill acquisition.

In the termination phase this scaffolding is gradually withdrawn and the relationship can effectively and purposely lose momentum and either dissolve completely or develop a new dynamic beyond the context of the mentoring relationship.

'Emotional labour'

This is a concept developed by the American sociologist Arlie Hochschild, who in 1983 published her study on the behaviour of flight attendants and argued that they used their emotions as part of their work and are required to display a particular emotional disposition regardless of whether or not it is in keeping with their own emotions. It has applied to healthcare by writers such as James (1989), usually to discuss practitioner–client interaction.

There are two broad aspects of emotional labour, the first being surface emotional labour and in this instance the worker has to manufacture and convey a sense of interest and feeling. The alternative is deep emotional labour where the worker has to change their subjective feelings to meet the objective needs of the organisation. The term has been broadened to refer to situations where emotions are involved and it captures much of the affectively based interaction between the health professional and the patient. Since time needs to be spent reassuring patients in the initial parts of a podiatric consultation either prior to or during a clinical management intervention and most professionals are socially skilled enough to do so automatically, the initial chat about the weather or holidays can be regarded as emotional labour.

This is an important concept within the context of mentorship and podiatric medicine, as it is useful to firstly consider what mentorship is not; and it is not a therapeutic alliance nor is it a social friendship. One of the dangers of one-to-one working is that a degree of friendship will arise and whilst this is not a bad thing it is important that clear boundaries and parameters of professional practice are established during the student's scheduled time on placement. The student is in the clinical setting to learn and the mentor is required to facilitate that process and assist the student to reflect on and develop their practice. Whilst issues arising from practice and client interaction are appropriate to discuss, personal issues and difficulties within the context of pastoral welfare are not and should be passed onto the relevant personnel, such as the course tutor.

Shakespeare and Webb (2008) from the findings of their qualitative research study discuss the emotional labour apparent in the mentorship relationship. They provide some interesting insights to mentorship and its functional processes. In addition to using emotional labour with clients the student also has to invest in emotional labour with their mentor as often when things go wrong it can be attributed to a lack of emotional labour, where the student has not invested energy in creating the correct impression with their mentor.

Impression management is an important idea and it is also one of the intangibles which the student learns as an integral part of the mentoring process. Newman (2009) gives a good definition of impression management as an 'act presenting a favourable public image of oneself so that others will form positive judgments' (p. 184). It is an aspect of professional life which most professionals instinctively get right but can on occasions be problematic. An example of this is the podiatry student who comes in covered in tattoos which may be a viable mechanism of self expression but which may be perceived as very off putting to a number of clients. Situational responses like this may need to be explored in the context of the mentorship relationship.

It is worth emphasising the affective component of the relationship, especially in situations where the mentor is working with the student in a one-to-one relationship where situations and issues which arise are inevitably more intense. The bulk of the literature comes from nursing and medical education where a number of people are involved and others are on hand to discuss the situation and provide support. It is important that if problems are encountered or the student is failing to achieve help is sought in a timely fashion before the dynamics of an effective relationship are allowed to falter.

'Communities of Practice'

This is a concept devised by Lave and Wenger, which emphasised the social aspect of learning.

Learning is a process in which people are incorporated into a community of practice, which surrounds a particular discipline or part of a discipline. Learning takes place both in a formal and in an informal sense, and the expectations of the profession, the ways in which theoretical ideas are transmitted in practice are all conveyed to the student. Lave and Wenger put this idea succinctly when they state it is not just learning from talk but learning to talk which is the key issue (Lave & Wenger, 1991, pp. 108–9).

As part of the clinical placement the student will learn not only about the formal aspects required by the curriculum but also will learn to work within the community of practice. This is an essential acknowledgement that a large part of the learning is about socialisation into the profession and how to conduct themselves in professional practice. This point has been already made in consideration of emotional labour and the student needs to develop those interactional skills which are an essential component of healthcare. The term tacit knowledge is often used but this goes wider than the human interactional skills and refers to those generic skills implicit in practice but which often are not articulated and can only be learned by engaging in professional practice. In the context of communities of practice it is the way that things are valued in that community, and can only be learned in practice. This is why the role of the mentor is invaluable in guiding the student.

Like many of the ideas which are explored in this chapter communities of practice are intangible. Whilst they may refer to a particular profession, they can also be used in connection with a less clearly defined population. Communities of practice may be the local community of podiatrists and the health professionals in the locality or the hospital. The theory emphasises learning as a social activity and the student can learn much from these wider communities both in a practical sense but also in the sense of learning what is acceptable practice and what the boundaries are of podiatric practice both in professional terms and in terms of what is acceptable within a particular locality.

Formative assessment

One of the roles of the mentor is as an assessor; this was briefly discussed earlier in the chapter. It may be in a very formal sense as the student is required to complete an assessment as part of their placement or informally as a mentor assisting with skill development. **Formative assessment** is an important concept and can be described as:

> *a moment of learning and students have to be active in their own assessment and to picture their own learning in light of what it means to get better*
>
> Black & William (1998, p. 29)

A clear distinction can be drawn between summative assessment, usually in the sense of completion or partial completion of an assignment, and assessment in the context of the ongoing learning process (Black & William, 1998). However, the basic principles are the same in both approaches. Black and William (1999) outline principles for successful assessment: effective feedback, active involvement of learners, adjustment of teaching to take account of assessment, recognising the effect assessment can have on the student and the need for self assessment by 'students'.

> Summative assessment is the making of a decision about the outcome of a course of study and about the progress of a learner. Formative assessment is concerned more precisely with diagnosis and establishment of the particular learning needs of students (Ecclestone, 1996)

Assessment can be a very powerful tool, which can greatly assist learning (Ecclestone, 1996; Black & William, 1998, 1999). However, several researchers identify that bad assessment can be a de-motivator and can have a negative effect both on the learner and on learning (for example, Ecclestone, 1996; Torrance, 1995). It is therefore important to ensure that the learning needs of students are diagnosed and established. On the basis of this an action plan can be developed building on strengths and addressing areas of deficiency.

Motivation

The purpose and function of a formative assessment scheme is to promote autonomy and enhance the motivation of students, in other words to make them self-directed learners. Motivation is generally taken to be both intrinsic and extrinsic whereby the student is motivated by factors both internal and external to themselves. The aim of the formative assessment scheme is to encourage motivation which is intrinsic so that the student will become motivated to learn and develop their skills in a productive and focused manner (Ecclestone, 2004). Howe (1999) discusses motivation and argues that achievement can be influenced by the extent the individual feels in control of the learning process. He maintains that the individual has an internal mechanism which he refers to as the *'locus of control'* (Rotter, 1975) which determines their interpretation of events. Causes of events can either be interpreted as due to internal or external factors. That is, in the case of assessment, the student can perceive the process is either controlled by external factors, the assessor, or that they have control over the learning process. The aim of formative assessment is to develop within the student an internal locus of control and ensure they have this sense of control over their learning.

Autonomy

Another approach to control of learning by the student is through the concept of autonomy. Ecclestone (2004) outlines a typology of autonomy and she maintains that there are three types: personal autonomy, procedural autonomy and critical autonomy. When the student gains personal autonomy they are able to effectively gauge their progress and establish ways in which they can achieve the intended outcomes of their programme of study. With procedural autonomy the student gains control over the practical or functional aspects of learning, that is he or she is able to manage and work within the system. In critical autonomy the student is expected to gain insights into their discipline and critically evaluate the state of their particular art.

Formative assessment schemes can promote the development of autonomy within the learner, certainly in procedural and personal autonomy, and ideally they will encourage the student to reflect on their work in such a way as to promote and encourage critical inquiry. Narrow standards or competency statements do little to promote critical autonomy; it is, therefore, important that standards are set which promote all ranges of autonomy.

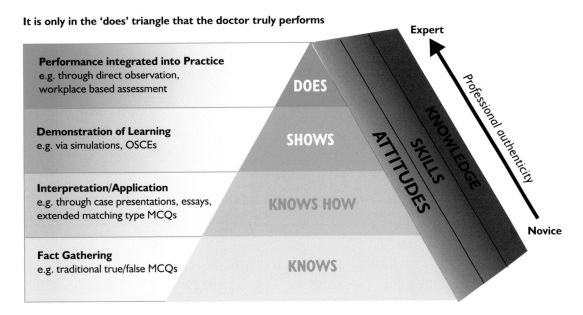

It is only in the 'does' triangle that the doctor truly performs

Performance integrated into Practice e.g. through direct observation, workplace based assessment	**DOES**
Demonstration of Learning e.g. via simulations, OSCEs	**SHOWS**
Interpretation/Application e.g. through case presentations, essays, extended matching type MCQs	**KNOWS HOW**
Fact Gathering e.g. traditional true/false MCQs	**KNOWS**

Figure 3.1: Miller's Prism of Clinical Competence (aka Miller's Pyramid)
Based on work by Miller G.E. The Assessment of Clinical Skills/Competence/Performance.
Acad. Med. 1990 65(9): 63–67. adapted by Drs. R Mehay & R. Burns. UK (Jan 2009)

The diagram by Miller (1990) (see figure 3.1), which is taken from the literature on medical education, provides a good framework for thinking about formative assessment. It highlights the interplay between knowledge, skills and attitudes which are integral to any situation where people are involved. There are the practical (psychomotor) skills which require manual dexterity and competence. The basis is the underpinning knowledge required to ensure the skill is not performed in a mechanical manner and integral to this is the correct attitude which ensures the patient is reassured, or put in another way the necessary emotional labour of the practitioner.

It also highlights the importance of ensuring that the student does incorporate skills, knowledge (cognition) and attitudes (affective interaction) in professional practice. It is worth remembering that educationally many students are prepared through the use of simulations and it only when in practice they actually apply their knowledge and skills in an integrative manner. The role of the mentor is essential in this process, as it is through feedback and discussion that personal and professional development can be facilitated.

Conclusion

The exploration of the role of the mentor in podiatric practice has revealed some of the underpinning theoretical ideas around the concept of mentorship. Constructionist approaches to learning (Vygotsky, 1978) were examined and the student was portrayed as someone actively engaged in their learning. The metaphor of scaffolding was used and this scaffolding could be gradually withdrawn as the learner developed. Ideas around 'Emotional Labour' (Hochschild, 1983), required in any form of interaction with people and applications both to client interaction and the student–mentor relationship were examined. Professional practice does not take place in a vacuum and induction into 'communities of practice' (Lave & Wenger, 1991) was explored. The chapter concludes with a consideration of formative assessment (Black & William, 1998) and the ways in which these principles underpin much of the mentorship relationship.

'Excellence is the result of making mundane all the actions that produce results... excellence which becomes second nature is what separates good swimmers from great ones.' (Chambliss, 1989). Chambliss was discussing the making of champion swimmers but the idea can be applied to mentorship and (to paraphrase) it is in assisting the student to make mundane all the actions that produce results...that achieves excellence in mentorship.

References

Ali, P.A. and Panther, W. (2008). 'Professional development and the role of mentorship' in *Nursing Standard*, **22**(42): 35–39.

Andrews, M. and Wallis, M. (1999). 'Mentorship in nursing: A literature review' in *Journal of Advanced Nursing*, **29**(1): 201–207.

Ausubel, D. (1963). *The Psychology of Meaningful Verbal Learning*. New York: Grune & Stratton.

Black, P. and William, D. (1998). 'Assessment and classroom learning' in *Assessment in Education*, **5**(1): 7–74.

Black, P. and William, D. (1999). *Assessment for Learning: Beyond the Black Box*, University of Cambridge School of Education: Assessment Reform Group. Available at: www.assessmentreformgroup.files.wordpress.com/2012/01/beyond_blackbox.pdf (accessed 13/06/12)

Cahill, H.A. (1996). 'A qualitative analysis of student nurses experiences of mentorship' in *Journal of Advanced Nursing*, **24**(4): 791–799.

Chambliss, D.R. (1989). 'The mundanity of excellence: An ethnographic report on stratification and olympic swimmers' in *Sociological Theory*, **7**(1): 70–86.

Ecclestone, K. (1996). *How to Assess the Vocational Curriculum (Vocational Education)*. London: Kogan.

Ecclestone, K. (2004). *Learning Autonomy in Post-16 Education*. London: Routledge.

Harden, R. and Crosby, J. (2000). *The good teacher is more than a lecturer - the twelve roles of the teacher*, University of Dundee: AMEE Medical Education Guide No. 20.

Hochschild, A.R. (1983). *The Managed Heart: Commercialization of Human Feeling*. Berkeley, CA: University of California Press.

Howe, M.J.A. (1999). *A Teacher's Guide to the Psychology of Learning*, Oxford: Blackwell.

James, N. (1989). 'Emotional labour: Skill and work in the social regulation of feelings' in *The Sociological Review*, **37**(1): 15–42.

Lave, J. and Wenger, E. (1991). *Situated Learning: Legitimate Peripheral Participation*, Cambridge: University of Cambridge Press.

Megginson, D. and Clutterbuck, D. (1995). *Mentoring in Action: A Practical Guide for Managers*, London: Sage.

Mezirow, J. (1991). *Transformative Dimensions of Adult Learning*. San Francisco: Jossey-Bass.

Miller, G.E. (1990). 'The assessment of clinical skills/competence/performance' in *Academic Medicine* **65**(9): [Suppl:S63-7].

Newman, D.M. (2009). *Sociology: Exploring the Architecture of Everyday Life*. Thousand Oaks, CA: Pine Forge Press.

Rotter, J. (1975). 'Some problems and misconceptions related to the construct of
internal versus external control of reinforcement' in *Journal of Consulting and Clinical Psychology*, **43**: 56–67.

Shakespeare, P. and Webb, C. (2008). 'Professional identity as a resource for talk: exploring the mentor–student relationship' in *Nursing Inquiry*, **15**(4): 270–279.

Spouse, J. (2001). 'Bridging theory and practice in the supervisory relationship: a sociocultural perspective' in *Journal of Advanced Nursing*, **33**(4): 512–522.

Torrance, H. (1995). *Evaluating Authentic Assessment: Problems and Possibilities in New Approaches to Assessment*. Buckingham: Open University Press.

Vygotsky, L.S. (1978). *Mind and Society: The Development of Higher Psychological Processes*, Cambridge, MA: Harvard University Press.

Wenger, E. (1998). *Communities of Practice: Learning, Meaning and Identity*. Cambridge: Cambridge University Press.

Chapter Four

Healthcare Organisations and Podiatry

Dr Alan M Borthwick, Professor Susan Nancarrow
and Associate Professor Rosalie Boyce

Contextualising the organisational-professional interface

Within contemporary healthcare, a broad, overarching network of healthcare organisations variously concerned with regulatory, legal and governance functions interfaces directly (and indirectly) with the profession of podiatry, informing and shaping its policy, practice and strategic direction. Some are concerned with broad issues relating to the quality and safety of professional services, such as the Care Quality Commission (CQC), and some with highly specific elements of professional practice, such as the use of medicines, as in the case of the Medicines and Healthcare Products Regulatory Agency (MHRA). Collectively they form a penumbra around the profession, ultimately linking it to the wider healthcare policy agenda. Operating in the interstices between these organisations, the healthcare professions seek to define their own aims and goals, and to maintain as high a degree of political, technical and economic autonomy as possible (Elston 1991; Hugman 1991; Freidson 2001). Structurally, professions establish their own representative organisations, which act to advance the collective interests of the membership, and constitute the professions' public face (Dagnall, 1995a; Dagnall, 1995b; Dagnall, 1995c; Boyce, 2006; Ackroyd *et al.*, 2007).

The relationship between the healthcare professions and the broader healthcare organisations within whose influence and remit they fall has been the object of attention within both sociology and organisational studies, and in this chapter we focus on the profession of podiatry as a case exemplar of the relationships between these authoritative bureaucratic organisations and the allied health professions (Boyce, 2006; Ackroyd *et al.*, 2007). In order to accurately contextualise the basis of these relationships, it is important to comment on the allied health professions within the hierarchy of the health division of labour (Larkin, 1983; Turner, 1985; Hugman, 1991).

For much of the twentieth century (and into the twenty-first century) medicine has occupied a hegemonic position within healthcare, exercising both social and cultural authority (Freidson, 1970b; Freidson, 1988; Willis, 1989; Freidson, 2001; Willis, 2006). Throughout much of that time, it has subjected the other, non-medical professions to one of three processes: **exclusion** (from mainstream, legitimate healthcare), **limitation** (to discrete areas of practice) or **subordination** (Turner, 1985; Turner, 1995). As a result, the allied health professions have sought to counter these strategies, and to engage in usurping tactics to advance their own interests and acquire and assert their own autonomy (Larson, 1977; Parkin, 1979; Larkin, 1983). Within this context, the relationship between the allied health professions and the organisations which surround them is dynamic and subject to constant change, influenced by shifting economic, political and social priorities (Harrison & Pollitt, 1994; Clarke, 2004; Sanders & Harrison, 2008). Central to this nexus is the balance between professional and organisational aims, and the transformative nature of alliances that are formed, dissolved and reformed over time (Currie *et al.*, 2009; Leicht *et al.*, 2009; Muzio & Kirkpatrick, 2011; Noordegraaf, 2011).

Podiatry and the organisational penumbra

In the case of podiatry, the relationship between the profession and the array of healthcare organisations with which it must interact is influenced by the broader political ideological and policy agenda, in turn shaped by wider concerns, such as recent workforce redesign initiatives aimed at addressing pressing demographic concerns (Cameron, 2003; Nancarrow & Borthwick, 2005). For example, following the inception of the Health Professions Council (HPC) in 2001, the profession was afforded a protected title in exchange for extended levels of public accountability and transparency (Borthwick, 2000b; Larkin, 2002). This accorded directly with the Blair government (1997–2008) mantra of 'rights and responsibilities', reflecting one of the underpinning ideological maxims informing the Third Way, espoused by New Labour, where legal and regulatory rights would be granted with the expectation and requirement that the profession(s) would accede to demands for greater accountability (Malin *et al.*, 2002). In turn, this stance reflected government concerns over patient safety issues (Kennedy, 2001).

Clear links exist between the professions, such as podiatry, and the institutional healthcare organisations that surround them; they reflect dynamic relationships that are symbiotic yet contradictory, stemming from the tensions between professional and bureaucratic objectives (Muzio & Kirkpatrick, 2011). Although the professional body undoubtedly sets the strategic direction of the profession, this is both modified and moulded by the limitations and opportunities presented by the broader policy agenda and enforced via legislation or regulation. In many instances these relationships are set within a national context, bound by national laws and regulatory requirements (Moran, 2002). Yet the globalisation of healthcare professions and organisations is increasingly evident, and is likely to play a greater role over time (Evetts, 2002; Jeffries & Evetts 2010). In this chapter, the relationships between healthcare professions and organisations are addressed both theoretically and empirically, drawing on two contemporary exemplars from within the field of podiatry. They are addressed as dynamic, co-dependent arrangements, comprising, on the one hand, the 'professional project' of the profession of podiatry (Larson, 1977), and on the other the policy imperatives of the organisations (Muzio & Kirkpatrick, 2011).

Healthcare organisations and professions: bureaucracy versus autonomy?

Theoretically, the relationships between the professions and those healthcare organisations within which (or for which) they increasingly operate are being steadily redefined. New Public Management reforms informed by neoliberal political ideologies have returned to the agenda as a result of both demographic and fiscal/economic concerns (Taylor-Gooby, 2011). Whereas some have suggested that the future for professions and professionalism is bleak, being eviscerated by the malign forces of 'managerial routinisation, technological commoditisation and cultural demystification' (Muzio & Ackroyd, 2005; Reed, 2007; Muzio & Kirkpatrick, 2011), most agree that the professions are rarely powerless to resist the encroachment of bureaucracy or the imposition of new regulatory requirements (Ackroyd, 1996; Muzio & Ackroyd, 2005; Ackroyd *et al.*, 2007; Scott, 2008). Indeed, professions may resist organisational demands, reverting to closure strategies or other exclusionary means of control, or may embrace new opportunities by 'moving into new markets, spaces and domains' (Muzio & Ackroyd, 2005; Thomas & Davies, 2005; Ackroyd *et al.*, 2007; Scott ,2008; Muzio & Kirkpatrick 2011). In the former instance, one of the most cogent concepts relevant to the relationships between podiatry and the broader arena of healthcare organisations is, arguably, Magili Larson's conceptual framework known as the '**professional project**' (Larson, 1977; Macdonald, 1995).

Professions, in attempting to further their aims and enhance their social, legal and financial standing, engage in activities to promote and advance the aims, but which require the endorsement of powerful social elites, such as the legislature, regulatory authorities, and the state authorities (such as the Department of Health) (Larson, 1977; Macdonald, 1995). Thus, these relationships are founded on a dynamic which is both potentially conflictual yet necessarily co-operative. Larkin (2002) detected a gradual but marked shift in the formerly secure, mutually beneficial arrangements of the '**medico-bureaucratic alliance**', a partnership between medicine and the state, with a more actively managed control. Certainly, demographic imperatives, fiscal constraints and rising public expectations have brought a sea change in the way the professions have been perceived and regulated, manifest in the reforms of both the Thatcher/Major era, and the modernising Blair government (Larkin, 2002; Nancarrow & Borthwick, 2005; Allsop, 2006; Dent, 2006). As a result, the profession of podiatry has become more accountable, transparent, open to challenge and strictly regulated, leading to shifting relationships with other healthcare organisations.

Adapting to bureaucratic challenges: a new professionalism?

However, the literature bears witness to the emergence of new countervailing strategies and identities, supporting the thesis that professions are dynamic and adaptable in the face of major bureaucratic challenges. Whether through recourse to 'restratification', separating a given profession into hierarchical tiers (Freidson, 2001;

Coburn, 2006), or acquiring new organisational, rather than professional, identities (Carmel, 2006), the capacity of professions to respond remains impressive and varied. Faced with organisational demands for performance appraisal, productivity objectives and accountability, professions may also reframe the discourse of professionalism and reconfigure professional identities in order to better fit corporate priorities (Cooper & Robson, 2006). Indeed, it is postulated that the tendency to depict professions and organisations as in direct opposition may in itself be flawed (Bourgeault *et al.*, 2011; Muzio & Kirkpatrick, 2011). Whereas the collegiality and autonomy of professionalism has been set against the bureaucracy of organisations, there is evidence to suggest that these two notions are not entirely incompatible and that, in any event, they lack historical accuracy (Bourgeault *et al.*, 2011). In addition, professions are thought to respond pragmatically to 'service realities' (Suddaby *et al.*, 2007; Noordegraaf & Schinkel, 2010; Noordegraaf, 2011). Certainly, the advent of managerialism in the UK NHS did impose new restrictions on professional freedom, and enabled non-professional (non-medical) managers to manage across professional boundaries, described as a 'non-negotiated order' (Cox, 1991). The logic of the market and of fiscal constraint, in reining in the excesses of a profligate and self-serving monopoly (as the medical profession was viewed), did involve conflicts between the professions and their employing organisations (Gabe *et al.*, 1994). However, in the UK at least, healthcare professions have, since the advent of the NHS, been integrated with, and dependent upon, those employing and regulating organisations. A range of advantages to the professions have been identified from the literature by Bourgeault *et al.,* (2011), including access to the bureaucratic institutions of education (universities), as well as career structures, tenure, access to financial resources and status. Yet, the ultimate goals of these healthcare organisations may conflict with the wishes of the professions.

In order to illustrate the complex knot which links key external healthcare organisations with the profession of podiatry, two contemporary exemplars are utilised. Each highlights the role played by relevant healthcare organisations in shaping the profession's destiny, and demonstrates the importance of aligning professional goals with the broader policy agenda in order to achieve advancement. In the first example, the acquisition of rights to prescribe medicines is used to demonstrate the convergence of organisational policy aims and professional aspirations. In the second, the dispute over the use of the title 'podiatric surgeon' draws attention to the dissonance in professional and organisational aims.

Prescribing of medicines: convergence in professional and organisational aims

In both the UK and Australia, the profession of podiatry has had a long history of access and administration rights to a limited range of medicines (Borthwick *et al.*, 2010). As the literature has demonstrated, acquiring even modest change in this arena has been problematic for those professions excluded from the list of 'approved prescribers' under the terms of the Medicines Act (1968) (Eaton & Webb, 1979; Gilbert, 1998; McCartney *et al.*, 1999; Taylor, 1999; Britten, 2001; Needle *et al.*, 2007). Freidson's assertion that the 'physician's right to diagnose, cut and prescribe' constituted the core of the medical profession's authority, and thus, by implication, were likely to be the three specific role domains most hotly contested in any jurisdictional dispute, proved prophetic (Freidson 1970b; Abbott 1988; Freidson 1988; Borthwick 2001a). Nevertheless, medical objections were unable to resist the flow of healthcare policy stemming from the pressing need for workforce flexibility and healthcare modernisation (Department of Health, 2000; Nancarrow & Borthwick, 2005; Department of Health, 2008a; Department of Health, 2008b).

With Ministerial support, the recommendations of the Crown report on the review of prescribing of medicines, advocating new categories of non-medical prescriber, were readily accepted by Government (Department of Health, 1999). Role and task transfer, central to the broader policy agenda seeking to address the impending demographic imperative, was viewed as essential, re-shaping the workforce and ensuring greater flexibility and thus service sustainability (Nancarrow & Borthwick, 2005). By 2005, professions such as podiatry, radiography and physiotherapy had become eligible for 'supplementary prescribing' status (Borthwick, 2008). Within a further three years, nursing, pharmacy and optometry had progressed to independent prescribing status (Latter *et al.*, 2010). As a further stage in the progress towards implementing the Crown report reforms (1999), the Department of Health established an AHP Prescribing Scoping Project, exploring the need for reform of existing mechanisms for access to medicines by allied health professions, including podiatry (Department of Health, 2009). It recommended that podiatry and physiotherapy be considered for independent prescribing rights. Although the prospect was greeted with medical disdain (Hawkes, 2010), the project proceeded, with Ministerial approval, through the necessary stages of public consultation. Presently (at the time of writing), the project is approaching the final stages of preparation for a submission to the Commission on Human Medicines.

Aligning goals: co-dependence or conformity?

Each stage in the process amply demonstrates the profession's dependence upon bureaucratic processes and institutions. Every facet of preparation has involved input from several healthcare organisations with governance, regulatory, legal and educational foci, addressing the outline curricular framework to inform educational programmes, an impact assessment, equality assessment, professional guidance, prescribing standards and competencies and so on. Implementation requires both regulatory (NHS regulations, professional regulation) and legislative change (amendments to the Medicines Act). At face value, it may seem as though this entire process is merely bureaucratic, and essentially procedural. In reality, it is a highly controversial issue which is contested – as the public consultation responses reveal – and it is dependent upon the support of these healthcare organisations which are in turn informed by the broader ideological and political environment.

As a case exemplar of the nature of the relationships between podiatry and the penumbra of healthcare organisations that surround it, the issue of prescribing highlights three key points which are critical to an understanding of the social, political and economic considerations that are instrumental in securing change. First, there is, of necessity, a web of different healthcare organisations involved in advancing initiatives such as enhanced prescribing for podiatry. Several healthcare organisations are required to ensure the necessary legislative change, regulatory approval, and re-alignment in educational programmes. The Department of Health, HPC, MHRA, Home Office, National Prescribing Centre, and professional bodies are all involved, as are, ultimately, the universities. Secondly, and critically, individual health professions such as podiatry are unable to advance and enact these developments in isolation; they are dependent upon access to external power resources, manifest as bureaucratic organisations. Thirdly, as this particular case illustrates, a convergence of professional and bureaucratic objectives is ultimately necessary to securing a successful outcome – indeed, it is a prerequisite.

Although central to the aims and goals of the professional project of podiatry, it would be disingenuous to suggest that prescribing rights could be achieved by the profession alone. Broader health policy goals will inevitably dictate the direction of change; if these converge with those of the professions, then there is a greater likelihood that the professions will succeed in attaining their desired outcomes. It is equally the case that a failure to achieve congruence between professional and organisational aims may lead to a failure to achieve the desired outcomes of the professions, which, in the case of podiatry, has so often been evident in the past (Larkin, 1983; Borthwick, 2001a).

Podiatric surgery: dissonance in professional and organisational aims

The practice of invasive foot surgery by non-medically qualified podiatrists has proven to be a deeply controversial and hotly contested issue, particularly in the UK and Australia (Borthwick, 2000a; Menz *et al.*, 2010). It is a major challenge to medical exclusivity in the arena of surgical practice, as well as a significant boundary encroachment into the role and task domains of the medical profession – most notably the specialty of orthopaedic surgery (Borthwick, 2000a; Borthwick, 2001a; Borthwick, 2001b; Borthwick, 2005). Nevertheless, in the era of GP fund holding, competitive tendering for contracts and internal managed markets, podiatric surgery in the UK grew to become an established feature of mainstream healthcare provision within England (Borthwick, 2000; Editorial, 1995). As an accessible, cost effective and clinically useful alternative to orthopaedic services, it provided an appealing option at a time when neoliberal, market based values dominated the political arena and suffused healthcare policy (Department of Health, 1994; Editorial, 1995).

During the period of healthcare marketisation and the introduction of managerialist reforms under successive Conservative governments, competition in the provision of healthcare services was adopted in a bid to improve efficiency and reduce costs (Ham, 2004). GPs were increasingly encouraged to act as business managers, purchasing services that provided the best value for money (Ham, 2004). By the early 1990s podiatric surgeons had become established as viable service providers for foot surgery, capable of competing with orthopaedic services for NHS and GP contracts (Editorial, 1995; Milsom, 1995). Under New Labour, the 'modernisation' of healthcare services offered further opportunities to challenge 'traditional ways of working', and enabled podiatric surgeons to offer flexible options and new pathways to match patient demand, expectation and choice (Department of Health, 2000; Helm & Ravi, 2003). Endorsed by the Department of Health, podiatric surgeons were granted title and pay levels commensurate with consultant grade positions under 'Agenda for Change', and the title was recognised in employment contracts, some of which were established as MC21 medical consultant contracts (Borthwick, 2000a; Department of Health, 2001b). Lord Hunt of King's Heath declared that 'the development of podiatric surgery is consistent with the Government's desire to end traditional demarcations which may inhibit the modernisation of services' (Lord Hunt of King's Heath, 2000). In contrast, hostile attitudes from orthopaedics were largely dismissed as monopolistic, entrenched in notions of medical exclusivity, and unsustainable in a modern healthcare service.

Under the earlier Conservative administrations, the adoption of market-oriented policies in the health services acted to encourage competitive practices and promote alternative providers of services, providing a potent policy direction which aligned neatly with professional aspirations in podiatry (as far as podiatric surgery was concerned). Successful integration of podiatric surgery into mainstream healthcare services was enabled by the broader policy agenda which promoted competition among providers of care who could demonstrate both clinical and cost effectiveness (Borthwick, 2000a). An alignment in professional and organisational objectives, at a given point in time, ensured progress, in spite of co-existing boundary disputes between the service providers of orthopaedics and podiatry. What is particularly useful in this case is that the convergence in professional and organisational aims altered over time, and in fact moved towards divergence, not as a result of a fundamental shift in healthcare policy, but because of an organisational challenge to professional autonomy, focused around public safety.

Throughout the period in which the provision of podiatric surgical services was accepted as a legitimate alternative option to orthopaedic foot care, in line with the dominant political ideology of neoliberalism, and subsequently through the period of healthcare modernisation encompassing and promoting workforce flexibility, medical opposition to podiatric surgery was viewed as essentially monopolistic and reactionary. Medical objection to the use by podiatrists of the titles of 'consultant', and 'podiatric surgeon' was largely dismissed as tribalism, and as a result, was never fully addressed or resolved (Hunter, 1994). Whilst use of the term 'consultant' by non-medically qualified health professionals became a widely accepted practice, and one incorporated into healthcare policies as part of New Labour's bid to modernise services, recruit greater numbers of allied health professionals, and establish career pathways in allied health (Department of Health, 2008a; Department of Health, 2008b), ambiguity continued to surround the use of the term 'podiatric surgeon'. Nevertheless, as long as the prevailing healthcare policies continued to promote workforce flexibility, cross boundary working and commissioning practices that emphasised cost and clinical effectiveness (that is, as long as podiatric surgical provision continued to meet organisational needs), then there was little need for organisational intervention. Increasingly, healthcare policy and organisational priorities were focused on patient experience and service provision; in each instance, podiatric surgery appeared to offer good value (Laxton, 1993; Hood *et al.*, 1994; Kilmartin, 2002; Helm & Ravi, 2003; Yates & Williamson, 2005).

The storm clouds gather: altruism in doubt?

More recently, however, the dispute around title re-emerged, but in a political climate in which the medical profession was no longer viewed as acting in a tribal and self-interested way, and where public *safety* became the central focus of concern (Allsop, 2006; Noordegraaf & Schinkel, 2010; Noordegraaf, 2011). As one of the central organisational priorities, patient safety, in line with the coalition government health policy agenda (again stressing market values, individual freedom and patient choice) prompted a reaction from both the Department of Health and government Health Ministers on the issue of the use of the title 'surgeon' by non-medically qualified surgeons. Instrumental in reigniting the controversy and in drawing a reaction from the Department of Health was the way in which the debate was played out in the public arena, via the media. Public involvement proved an essential ingredient in persuading the Department to challenge the profession's autonomy, and attempt to exercise its bureaucratic authority to effect a change in title.

What was, at an earlier stage, an ambiguity which did not require action now appeared to merit direct intervention. At stake was the use of the title 'podiatric surgeon', which, it was contended, breached the terms of the Medical Act (1983), which stipulated that '*any person who wilfully and falsely pretends to be or takes or uses the name or title of physician, doctor of medicine, licentiate in medicine and surgery, bachelor of medicine, surgeon, general practitioner or apothecary, or any name, title, addition or description implying that he is...*' would be liable to prosecution. There were two elements to the argument. First, adoption of the title by podiatrists practising foot surgery could be construed as a breach of the Act by virtue of the restrictions placed by it on the use of the term 'surgeon'. Second, continuing to use the title when actively aware that doing so may be a breach of the Medical Act could be construed as a 'wilful and false' use of the title. Underpinning both points was a concern that use of the title would mislead the public into assuming that the bearer of such a title would be medically qualified.

What, then, had changed? It was well known that the issue of the legality of the title 'podiatric surgeon' had been questioned several times over the previous twenty years, with conflicting legal advice offered on all sides, but without firm resolution (Borthwick, 2000a). It was not the law or its possible interpretation that had fundamentally changed – recent legal evaluations referred to the same precedents in case law as had earlier considerations – it was simply that, by 2010, the issue had become a public interest issue, and that medical objections were no longer perceived as acts of professional self-interest, but taken to be genuine concerns for public safety. A litany of public safety incidents in healthcare – from the Harold Shipman case to the Bristol Inquiry – had sensitised Government to the risk of damaging scandals (Kennedy, 2001; Allsop, 2006; Noordegraaf & Schinkel, 2010; Noordegraaf, 2011).

Initial convergence in organisational policy and professional aims

Podiatric surgery had, by 2001, become an accepted fact of NHS provision, to the extent that the Royal College of Surgeons of Edinburgh, at the instigation of the Scottish Executive (Scottish Government), had undertaken to enter into discussions with the Society of Chiropodists and Podiatrists with a view to establishing a jointly recognised training programme in foot surgery, under the auspices of the Royal College of Surgeons of Edinburgh. At that time there were no consultant podiatric surgeons practising in Scotland, and the Scottish government was clearly looking to adopt the English model of foot surgical provision. Whilst there were 'many concerns' expressed by the Royal College, it was reported that 'it seemed inevitable that podiatrists would be allowed to work in the NHS in Scotland and it would, thus, be best to supervise this development rather than be excluded' (Royal College of Surgeons of Edinburgh, 2001). Establishing a joint diploma in podiatric surgery would, it was asserted, 'ensure that those podiatrists were not autonomous but worked in multi-disciplinary teams' (Royal College of Surgeons of Edinburgh, 2001). By 2002, a Memorandum of Understanding had been signed between the two bodies, and had the apparent support of the British Orthopaedic Association. At more or less the same time, the Department of Health had issued a letter confirming approval by the Secretary of State for Health for alterations to be made to remuneration and conditions of service for professions allied to medicine in recognition of new 'consultant' posts, in line with the policy outlined in the NHS Plan (Department of Health, 2001a; Department of Health, 2001b). However, the British Orthopaedic Association, although supportive of the Edinburgh initiative, continued to object to the use of the title 'consultant podiatric surgeon'. Whilst willing to acknowledge podiatric surgeons as independent practitioners (albeit to a limited extent: 'restricted to the toes'), and to recognise that the term 'consultant' was not a protected title, and even that the term 'surgeon' could be 'variously applied', the BOA President considered its use by podiatrists to be misleading.

The intervention of the media: divergence in organisational policy and professional aims

In August 2004, the first of a trail of media reports focusing on podiatric surgery began to enter the public arena. It claimed that the British Orthopaedic Trainee's Association (an organisation within the British Orthopaedic Association) had 'declared open war' on podiatric surgeons, claiming that they had 'no medical qualifications at all'. At the heart of the article was the assertion that the public was being 'deceived', citing a survey carried out by an orthopaedic specialist registrar which canvassed the views of members of the public. Ninety-five per cent were said to have believed that a consultant podiatric surgeon was medically qualified. In it, the President of the BOA was cited as asserting that 'we have repeatedly complained, but we get no help from the General Medical Council, and absolutely none from the Department of Health', because, it was claimed, 'the Department of Health thinks podiatric surgeons are wonderful because they are quick to train, cheap, and take patients off orthopaedic waiting lists' (Hawkes, 2004). Thus, at the start of the media interest in the topic, it was clear that broader healthcare policy organisational objectives did not conflict with the professional aspirations of podiatry (Editorial, 2002). Indeed, the article itself may have been prompted by a wider concern within orthopaedics that the Department of Health was considering plans to appoint a series of podiatric consultants to run orthopaedic triage clinics, thus controlling orthopaedic referral streams. At this point, medical objections were, therefore, likely to have been viewed as reactionary and as a form of resistance to workforce redesign measures. In the resulting 'letters to the editor', replies from medical professionals tended to reflect this point (Essex, 2004; Loughran, 2004; Magee, 2004). Within weeks, another two newspaper articles appeared, each raising similar concerns and citing similar sources (Crompton, 2004; Goldacre, 2004). By 2008, *The Telegraph* had entered the debate, airing the views of an orthopaedic surgeon claiming that podiatric surgeons were 'confusing' patients (Devlin, 2008), and in 2009 *The Times* had returned to the topic, publishing an article questioning the competence of podiatrists to practice surgery (Davies, 2009). Indeed, the Patient Liaison Group of the Royal College of Surgeons had expressed general concerns about the titles of 'non-medically qualified practitioners' as early as 2005 (Getty, 2001), bringing direct patient concerns to the fore, although it was not until 2010 that its response to the HPC consultation on registering titles for podiatric surgeons gave it a public platform.

Enter the BBC: broadening the debate, escalating the concern

A significant transition in alignment between professional and organisational aims was signalled by a BBC London television programme devoted to the issue of podiatric surgery, broadcast on 7 December 2009 (Cavell, 2009). Central to the report was the assertion that patients were being confused and wilfully misled by podiatrists, and it attempted to draw negative comparisons between the training of podiatric and orthopaedic surgeons. For the first time, the programme reported an expression of concern by the Department of Health about the use of the title 'surgeon' by podiatrists. It also drew a response from the Health Professions Council, which assured the BBC it would 'review' the use of title by podiatrists, and also claimed that a London MP was seeking to raise the matter in Parliament (Cavell, 2009). Another article, citing similar content and claiming as misleading the tendency to combine the two terms 'consultant' and 'surgeon', in a novel twist to the saga, was published in *The Telegraph* (Getty, 2010). The Department of Health contacted the Society of Chiropodists and Podiatrists in 2010 to express its concern, and even to suggest alternative titles that the Department would be prepared to accept. At present, the Faculty of Podiatric Surgery is shortly to consider the issue of title again, with a view to finding a final resolution to the dispute. What is abundantly clear is that, unlike earlier organisational responses to these arguments, public safety issues were at the heart of Departmental concerns, and prompted a sea change in attitudes at the Department of Health and among the Health Ministers, forcing the profession to reconsider its position on the use of titles. What had previously been perceived as an inter-professional dispute over task domains now touched on areas of Government concern, thus creating a misalignment in organisational and professional aims. Critical to the shift in attitude was the advent of a new political climate, defined in the literature as a 'risk' culture (Lupton, 1999), raising fears about the politically damaging consequences of further revelations that might discredit health services (Millenson, 2002; Allsop, 2006; Waring & Bishop, 2011). These concerns were amplified directly by the media attention. As Noordegraaf (2011) cogently noted, 'the media like to focus on specific cases and particularly incidents, in order to define risk and show mistreatment and service failure'.

Another relevant policy shift which lent itself to the arguments being aimed at podiatric surgeons was the drive towards multi-professionalism (Clavering & McLaughlin, 2007; Reynolds, 2007; Huotari, 2008; Edwards *et al.*, 2009). Increasingly healthcare has been viewed, within the context of workforce redesign and flexibility, as addressing complex social and healthcare problems – so called 'multi-problems' (Huotari, 2008) – raising pressure on inter-professional teams, and demanding multi-disciplinary co-operation and multi-agency working (Nancarrow & Borthwick 2005; Currie *et al.*, 2009). Thus, orthopaedic calls for ascendancy in a co-operative, collaborative relationship appeared consistent with broader health policy aims and may, therefore, need to be viewed with caution by the podiatry profession in future (Macnicol, 2007).

Conclusions

As these two case exemplars illustrate, autonomous healthcare professions are, nevertheless, subject to the overarching influence and authority of healthcare organisations such as the Department of Health. Large, powerful, bureaucratic organisations are increasingly important as providers of healthcare, utilising the skills and knowledge of professionals, yet exercising power over them. In a form of symbiosis, they provide stability and resources to the professions, and in return access and deploy their services. Yet the professions have not quite succumbed to proletarianisation or deprofessionalisation as passive victims, appearing to retain some potency in the face of bureaucratic control. Professional projects may still be advanced, but are only likely to succeed where they align with the broader policy objectives of the organisations within whose shadow they work.

References

Abbott, A. (1988). *The System of Professions – An Essay on the Division of Expert Labour.* Chicago: University of Chicago Press.

Ackroyd, S. (1996). 'Organizations contra organizations: professions and organizational change in the United Kingdom' in *Organization Studies*, **17**(4): 599–621.

Ackroyd, S., Kirkpatrick, I. and Walker, R.M. (2007). 'Public management reform in the UK and its consequences for professional organisation: a comparative analysis' in *Public Administration*, **85**(1): 9–26.

Allsop, J. (2006). 'Regaining trust in medicine' in *Current Sociology*, **54**(4): 621–636.

Borthwick, A. (2000a). 'Challenging medicine: the case of podiatric surgery' in *Work, Employment and Society,* **14**(2): 369–383.

Borthwick, A. (2000b). 'Podiatry and the state: Occupational closure strategies since 1960' in *British Journal of Podiatry*, **3**(1): 13–20.

Borthwick, A. (2001a). 'Drug prescribing in podiatry: Radicalism or tokenism?' in *British Journal of Podiatry*, **4**(2): 56–64.

Borthwick, A. (2001b). 'Occupational imperialism at work: the case of podiatric purgery' in *British Journal of Podiatry*, **4**(3): 70–79.

Borthwick, A., Short, A., Nancarrow, S.A. and Boyce, R. (2010). 'Non-medical prescribing in Australasia and the UK: the case of podiatry' in *Journal of Foot and Ankle Research*, **3**(1).

Borthwick, A.M. (2005). ' "In the beginning": Local anaesthesia and the Croydon Postgraduate Group' in *British Journal of Podiatry*, **8**(3): 87–94.

Borthwick, A.M. (2008). 'Professions allied to medicine and prescribing' in *Non-Medical Prescribing – Multi-disciplinary Perspectives*. P. Nolan and E. Bradley, Cambridge: Cambridge University Press: pp. 133–164.

Bourgeault, I., Hirshkorn, K. and Sainsaulieu, I. (2011). 'Relations between professions and organisations: more fully considering the role of the client' in *Professions and Professionalism*, **1**(1): 67–86.

Boyce, R. (2006). 'Emerging from the shadow of medicine: allied health as a "profession community" subculture' in *Health Sociology Review*, **15**(5): 520–533.

Britten, N. (2001). 'Prescribing and the defence of clinical autonomy' in *Sociology of Health & Illness*, **23**(4): 478–496.

Cameron, A. and Masterson, A. (2003). 'Reconfiguring the clinical workforce' in *The Future Health Workforce*. C. Davies (ed). Basingstoke: Palgrave Macmillan: pp. 68–86.

Carmel, S. (2006). 'Boundaries obscured and boundaries reinforced: incorporation as a strategy of occupational enhancement for intensive care' in *Sociology of Health and Illness*, **28**(2): 154–177.

Cavell, A. (2009). 'Concern over unregulated surgeons.' BBC London News (Monday, 7 December 2009). Available at: news.bbc.co.uk/local/london/low/tv_and_radio/newsid_8400000/8400189.stm (accessed 17/06/12).

Clarke, J. (2004). 'Dissolving the public realm? The logics and limits of neo-liberalism' in *Journal of Social Policy*, **33**(1): 27–48.

Clavering, E. and McLaughlin, J. (2007). 'Crossing multidisciplinary divides: Exploring professional hierarchies and boundaries in focus groups' in *Qualitative Health Research*, **17**(3): 400–410.

Coburn, D. (2006). 'Medical dominance then and now: critical reflections' in *Health Sociology Review*, **15**(5): 432–443.

Cooper, D. and Robson, K. (2006). 'Accounting, professions and regulation: locating the sites of professionalisation' in *Accounting, Organizations and Society*, **31**(4/5): 415–444.

Cox, D. (1991). 'Health service management – a sociological view: Griffiths and the non-negotiated order of the hospital' in *The Sociology of the Health Service*. J. Gabe, M. Calnan and M. Bury, eds. London: Routledge.

Crompton, S. (2004). 'Who's who in hospital?' in *The Times*, 4 September.

Currie, G., Finn, R. and Martin, G. (2009). 'Professional competition and modernizing the clinical workforce in the NHS' in *Work, Employment and Society*, **23**(2): 267–284.

Dagnall, J. (1995a). 'The origins of the Society of Chiropodists and Podiatrists and its history 1945–1995 (Part 1).' in *Journal of British Podiatric Medicine*, **50**(9): 135–141.

Dagnall, J. (1995b). 'The origins of the Society of Chiropodists and Podiatrists 1945–1995 (Part 2).' in *Journal of British Podiatric Medicine*, **50**(10): 151–156.

Dagnall, J. (1995c). 'The origins of the Society of Chiropodists and Podiatrists 1945-1995 (Part 3).' in *Journal of British Podiatric Medicine*, **50**(11): 174–180.

Davies, M. (2009). 'Doctor, doctor, my foot pain won't go away' in *The Times*, 7 February.

Dent, M. (2006). 'Disciplining the medical profession? Implications of patient choice for medical dominance' in *Health Sociology Review*, **15**(5): 458–468.

Department of Health (1994). *Feet First – Report of the Joint Department of Health and NHS Chiropody Task Force*. London: The Stationery Office.

Department of Health (1999). *Final Report of the Review of Prescribing, Supply and Administration of Medicines (The Crown Report)*. London: The Stationery Office.

Department of Health (2000). *The NHS Plan*. London: The Stationery Office.

Department of Health (2001a). *The NHS Plan – A Plan for Investment, A Plan for Reform*. London: The Stationery Office.

Department of Health (2001b). Arrangements for consultant posts for staff covered by the Professions Allied to Medicine PT "A" Whitley Council Advance Letter PAM (PTA) 2/2001.

Department of Health (2008a). *Framing the Contribution of the Allied Health Professionals: Delivering High-quality Healthcare*. London: The Stationery Office.

Department of Health (2008b). *Modernising Allied Health Professions (AHP) Careers: A Competence Based Career Framework*. London: The Stationery Office.

Department of Health (2009). *Allied Health Professions Prescribing and Medicines Supply Mechanisms Scoping Project Report*. London: The Stationery Office.

Devlin, K. (2008). 'Podiatrists confuse patients by calling themselves surgeons' in *The Telegraph*. London. Available at: www.telegraph.co.uk/health/3086093/Podiatrists-confuse-patients-by-calling-themselves-surgeons.html# (accessed 17/06/12).

Eaton, G. and Webb, B. (1979). 'Boundary encroachment: pharmacists in the clinical setting' in *Sociology of Health & Illness*, **1**(1): 69–89.

Editorial (1995). 'GPs Praise Podiatry' in *General Practitioner*, 24 February.

Editorial (2002). 'Chiropody, podiatry and orthopaedics' in *Foot and Ankle Surgery*, **8**(2): 83.

Edwards, A., Daniels, H., Gallagher, T., Leadbetter, J. and Warmington, P. (2009). *Improving Inter-professional Collaborations: Multi-agency Working for Children's Wellbeing*. London: Routledge.

Elston, M. (1991). 'The politics of professional power: medicine in a changing health service' in *The Sociology of the Health Service*. J. Gabe, M. Calnan and M. Bury, eds. London: Routledge.

Essex, N. (2004). 'Position of consultants in the NHS?' in *The Times*, letters to the Editor, 6 September: 17.

Evetts, J. (2002). 'New directions in state and international professional occupations: discretionary decision making and acquired regulation' in *Work, Employment and Society*, **16**(2): 341–353.

Freidson, E. (1970). *Professional Dominance: The Social Structure of Medical Care*. New York: Atherton Press.

Freidson, E. (1988). *Profession of Medicine – A Study of the Sociology of Applied Knowledge*. Chicago: University of Chicago Press.

Freidson, E. (2001). *Professionalism: The Third Logic*. Oxford: Oxford University Press.

Gabe, J. and Kelleher, D. (1994). *Challenging Medicine*. London: Routledge.

Getty, J. (2007). 'The President ex Cathedra' in *Newsletter of the British Orthopaedic Association* Spring(35): 1–2.

Getty, J. (2010). 'Medical job titles: what's in a name?' *The Telegraph*. London. 13t October. Available at: www.telegraph.co.uk/health/8062112/Medical-job-titles-whats-in-a-name.html (accessed 17/06/12).

Gilbert, L. (1998). 'Pharmacy's attempts to extend its role: a case study in South Africa' in *Social Science in Medicine*, **47**(2): 153–164.

Goldacre, B. (2004). 'It's all in a title.' *The Guardian*. London. 16 September. Available at: www.guardian.co.uk/science/2004/sep/16/badscience.research (accessed 17/06/12).

Ham, C. (2004). *Health Policy in Britain*. Basingstoke: Palgrave Macmillan.

Harrison, S. and Pollitt, C. (1994). *Controlling Health Professionals: The Future of Work and Organization in the NHS (State of Health)*. Buckingham: Open University Press.

Hawkes, N. (2004). ' "Consultants" treading on doctors' toes' in *The Times*, 30 August: 15.

Hawkes, N. (2010). 'Handing over the prescription pad.' in *British Medical Journal*, **340**: 73–75.

Helm, R. and Ravi, K. (2003). 'Podiatric surgery and orthopaedic surgery: a customer satisfaction survey of general practitioners' in *The Foot*, **13**: 53–54.

Hood, I., Kilmartin, T. and Tollafield, D. (1994). 'The effect of podiatric day care surgery on the need for National Health Service chiropody treatment' in *The Foot* **4**(3): 155–158.

Hugman, R. (1991). *Power in Caring Professions*. Basingstoke: Macmillan.

Hunter, D. (1994). 'From tribalism to corporatism: The managerial challenge to medical dominance,' in *Challenging Medicine*. J. Gabe, and G. Williams eds. London: Routledge.

Huotari, R. (2008). 'Development of collaboration in multiproblem cases: some possibilities and challenges' in *Journal of Social Work*, **8**(1): 83–98.

Jeffries, D. and Evetts, J. (2010). 'Approaches to the international recognition of professional qualifications in engineering and the sciences' in *European Journal of Engineering Education*, **25**(1): 99–107.

Kennedy, I. (2001). *Learning from Bristol – The Report of the Public Inquiry into childrens' heart surgery at the Bristol Royal Infirmary 1984-1995*, London: The Stationery Office.

Kilmartin, T. (2002). 'Podiatric surgery in a community Trust: a review of activity, surgical outcomes, complications and patient satisfaction over a 4 year period' in *The Foot*, **11**: 218–227.

Kilmartin, T. (2002). 'Revision of failed foot surgery: a critical analysis' in *Journal of Foot and Ankle Surgery*, **41**(5): 309–315.

Larkin, G. (1983). *Occupational Monopoly and Modern Medicine*. London: Tavistock.

Larkin, G. (2002). 'Regulating the professions allied to medicine' in *Regulating the Health Professions*. J. Allsop and M. Saks, eds. London: Sage.

Larson, M. (1977). *The Rise of Professionalism – A Sociological Analysis*. Berkeley: University of California Press.

Latter, S., Blenkinsop, A., Smith, A., Chapman, S., Tinelli, M., Gerard, K., Little, P., Celino, N., Granby, T., Nicholls, P. and Dorer, G.. (2010). *Evaluation of Nurse and Pharmacy Independent Prescribing*. London: The Stationery Office.

Leicht, K., Walter, T., Sainsaulieu, I. and Davies, S. (2009). 'New public management and new professionalism across nations and contexts' in *Current Sociology*, **57**(4): 581–605.

Lord Hunt of King's Heath (2000). 'Podiatric Surgery.' Hansard 15 March: Column WA213.

Loughran, C.(2004). 'Position of consultants in the NHS' in *The Times*, letters to the Editor, 6 September: 17.

Lupton, D. (1999). *Risk*. London: Routledge.

Macdonald, K. (1995). *The Sociology of the Professions*. London: Sage.

Macnicol, M. (2007). 'The President reports…' in *Newsletter of the British Orthopaedic Association*, 26: 1–2.

Magee, P. (2004). 'Whitehall control of consultants' in *The Times*, letters to the Editor, 4 September: 25

Malin, N., Wilmot, S. and Manthorpe, J. (2002). *Key Concepts and Debates in Health and Social Care*. Maidenhead: Open University Press.

McCartney, W., Tyrer, S. Brazier, M. and Prayle, D. (1999). 'Nurse prescribing: Radicalism or tokenism?' in *Journal of Advanced Nursing*, **29**(2): 348–354.

Medical Act (1983). General Medical Council.
Available at: www.gmc-uk.org/about/legislation/medical-act.asp (accessed 26/06/12).

Menz, H., Borthwick, A., Potter, M., Landorf, K. and Munteau, S. (2010). ' "Foot" and "surgeon": a tale of two definitions' in *Journal of Foot and Ankle Research*, **3**(30).

Millenson, M. (2002). 'Pushing the profession: How the news media turned patient safety into a priority' in *Quality and Safety in Health Care*, **11**(1): 57–63.

Milsom, P. (1995). 'Foot surgery: the podiatric option' in *The Practitioner*, **239**: 396–402.

Moran, M. (2002). 'The health professions in international perspective' in *Regulating the Health Professions*. J. Allsop and M. Saks (eds). London: Sage.

Muzio, D. and Ackroyd, S. (2005). 'On the consequences of defensive professionalism: the transformation of the legal labour process' in *Journal of Law and Society*, **32**(4): 615–642.

Muzio, D. and Kirkpatrick, I. (2011). 'Professions and organisations – a conceptual framework' in *Current Sociology*, 59(4): 380–405.

Nancarrow, S. and Borthwick, A. (2005). 'Dynamic professional boundaries in the healthcare workforce' in *Sociology of Health & Illness*, **27**(7): 897–919.

Needle, J., Lawrenson, J. G., and Petchley, R. (2007). *Scope and Therapeutic Practice: A Survey of UK Optometrists: a report prepared for the College of Optometrists*. London: City of London University.

Noordegraaf, M. (2011). 'Risky business: how professionals and professional fields (must) deal with organizational issues' in *Organization Studies,* **32**(10): 1349–1371.

Noordegraaf, M. and Schinkel, W. (2010). 'Professional capital contested: A Bourdieusian analysis of conflicts between professionals and managers' in *Comparative Sociology*, **10**(1): 1–29.

Parkin, F. (1979). *Marxism and Class Theory: A Bourgeois Critique*. London: Tavistock.

Reed, M. (2007). 'Engineers of human souls, faceless technocrats or merchants of morality? Changing professional forms and identities in the face of neoliberal reforms' in *Human Resource Management: ethics and employment*. A. Pinnington, R. Macklin and T. Campbell (eds). Oxford: Oxford University Press.

Reynolds, J. (2007). 'Discourses of inter-professionalism' in *British Journal of Social Work*, **37**(3): 441–457.

Royal College of Surgeons of Edinburgh (2001). Minutes of meeting of the Council of the College, 9 November.

Sanders, T. and Harrison, S. (2008). 'Professional legitimacy claims in the multidisciplinary workplace: The case of heart failure care' in *Sociology of Health and Illness*, **30**(2): 289–308.

Scott, W. (2008). 'Lords of the dance: Professionals as institutional agents' in *Organization Studies*, **29**(2): 219–238.

Suddaby, R., Cooper, C. and Greenwood, R. (2007). 'Transnational regulation of professional services: Governance dynamics of field level organizational change' in *Accounting, Organizations and Society*, **32**(4/5): 333–362.

Taylor-Gooby, P. (2011). 'Root and branch restructuring to achieve major cuts: the social policy programme of the 2010 UK Coalition Government' in *Social Policy and Administration*, **46**(1): pp. 61–82.

Taylor, R. (1999). 'Partnerships or power struggle? The Crown review of prescribing' in *British Journal of General Practice*, **49**(442): 340–341.

Thomas, R. and Davies, A. (2005). 'Theorizing the micro-politics of resistance: New public management and managerial identities in the UK public services' in *Organization Studies*, **26**(5): 683–706.

Turner, B. (1985). 'Knowledge, skill and occupational strategy: the professionalisation of paramedical groups' in *Community Health Studies*, **9**(1): 38–47.

Turner, B. (1995). *Medical Power and Social Knowledge*. London: Sage.

Waring, J. and Bishop, S. (2011). 'Healthcare identities at the crossroads of service modernisation: the transfer of NHS clinicians to the independent sector?' in *Sociology of Health and Illness*, **33**(5): 661–676.

Willis, E. (1989). *Medical Dominance: The Division of Labour in Australian Healthcare* (2nd ed.) London: George Allen and Unwin.

Willis, E. (2006). 'Introduction: taking stock of medical dominance' in *Health Sociology Review*, **15**(5): 421–431.

Yates, B. and Williamson, D. (2008). 'Integration of podiatric surgery within an orthopaedic department: an audit of patient satisfaction' in *Journal of Bone and Joint Surgery*, 90-B (Supplement II): 230.

Chapter Five

Management and Leadership for Podiatry

Gez Bevan

Framing Management and Leadership in Podiatry

Whilst the healthcare literature and healthcare systems are no strangers to the concepts of management and leadership, applying this intelligently to podiatry is a challenge. This in itself can be argued to be a significant feature, that within podiatry the literature and evidence relating to management and leadership has been relatively limited. More recently the issue has been how this can be addressed or redressed. In addition these issues cannot be divorced from the nature and scope of the healthcare economy, both in the UK and elsewhere.

The relative ease with which podiatric services can be acquired through private practice can be argued to be one of the significant factors relating to management and leadership in that for a very long time podiatry remained a disparate profession which operated in some cases in complete isolation from clinical governance structures. Lone practitioner status was, and to a great extent still is, commonplace and can be seen to exacerbate this issue.

In contextualising this, data from the UK Health Professions Council (HPC 2011) records the number of podiatrists/chiropodists registered with the HPC, as being marginally over 12,700 in October 2011. The HPC themselves refer to both chiropodists and podiatrists in the same part of the register and at a headline level it is not possible to distinguish between the two or even whether the HPC make a distinction between the two. Whether the use of the term podiatrist or chiropodist is descriptive, historic or representative of qualification and level of education is still open to question in this context. It is also true that there is a multiplicity of occupational groups registered with the HPC and that the register spans an enormous range, from degree qualified clinical scientists through to non-degree qualified technicians or dispensing technicians. The extent to which their practice brings them into close proximity to patients and whether they are autonomous in their practice also varies significantly.

When considered against other comparable occupations, (physiotherapists, occupational therapists and biomedical scientists) podiatry/chiropody represents the smallest group, both in terms of those historically registered with the precursor to the HPC, the Council for Professions Supplementary to Medicine (from 1967 until the transfer of statutory regulation to the HPC in 2004) and those currently registered with the HPC.

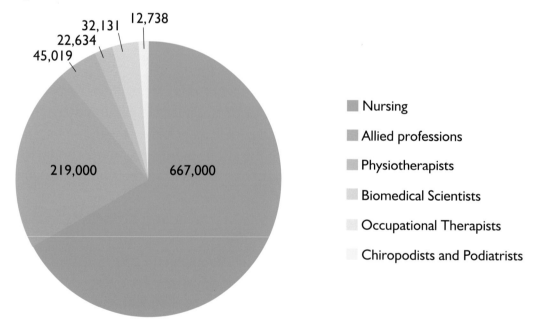

Figure 5.1: Numbers of selected professionals registered with their regulatory body in 2011

(Nursing - registered with the Nursing & Midwifery Council (NMC). All others with the Health Professions Council (HPC))

(Source: NMC 2011 and HPC 2011)

The loose nature of statutory registration from 1967 for podiatrists means that, though there was not a strict register, numbers can be given for those in practice or eligible to practise yielding an 'effective register'.

As with other regulatory bodies such as the Nursing and Midwifery Council (NMC) the early registers often contained names of those who were no longer practising or were deceased and a positive statement needed to be made in order for someone's name to be removed. Annual registration update has been a significant improvement in being able to produce data; as a result it is really only by around 2004 when the HPC became the statutory regulator for podiatrists that the data becomes more reliable. It can be argued that statutory registration with a single regulatory body has been beneficial for recruitment and retention in the profession.

Defining management and leadership

The relationship between knowledge and organisation is a good starting point from which to try to define management. In his earlier works Rousseau makes this point and identifies that knowledge of the human resources within organisations is the most significant tool available.

> *A real knowledge of things may be a good thing in itself, but the knowledge of men and their opinions is better, for in human society man is the chief tool of man, and the wisest man is he who best knows the use of this tool*
>
> *(Rousseau, 1972, p. 149)*

Drucker, although focusing on industry, industrial scale production and the relationship of people to that process, pursued this further and identified a clear synergy between knowledge and its use to the betterment of the end result.

> *Supplying knowledge to find out how existing knowledge can best be applied to produce results is, in effect, what we mean by management.*
>
> *(Drucker, 1993, p. 42)*

And so, whilst not exhaustive, it can be argued that within healthcare and in these circumstances within podiatry, successful management relies upon a clear relationship between knowing (knowledge) and doing (practice) which is the application of the knowledge to produce results, i.e. deliver or improve care. In essence the effective management of clinical events relies upon understanding and applying the knowledge, the evidence, in order to establish evidence-based practice.

Hartley and Benington (2010) make the observation that essentially management alone had, until recently, been argued to be the means by which healthcare organisations could be improved but that there has been a change in focus to that of leadership. Kotter (1990) argues that if management is about getting things done, by way of planning, organising and the effective use of resources, leadership is visionary and entails charting the course to be followed, essentially arguing that good leadership is essential before anything can be implemented (or managed). Storey (2004) identifies several factors which allow management and leadership to be defined, but also differentiated from each other.

Management	Leadership
● Attention to process and procedure	● Wider picture, a global perspective
● Maintaining status quo	● Challenging in order to effect change
● Monitor and control	● Enable and empower
● Putting into action (transacting)	● Transforming

Whilst a useful framework from which to be able to define and differentiate (if indeed differentiation is required) there is the risk that this becomes divisive with the net result being that differentiating management and leadership in this way inadvertently pits one against the other and creates a value-based judgement along the lines of 'leadership is good' and 'management is bad'. The reality, as Yukl (2006) argues, is that one is essential for the other and that in order to implement change and for this to be effective the skills of leadership are essential.

… success as a manager…involves leading…

(Yukl, 2006, p.6)

Differing management styles within podiatry, in relation to NHS reforms, were explored by Blakeman (2003) and in particular the relationship between professional identity and style of management. The most significant observation was that managers from 'within', i.e. drawn from the same professional group, demonstrated greater resentment around increased monitoring of activity and expectation that services could be extended and podiatric work undertaken by others, which was felt to be at odds with the requirements of their regulatory framework. In contrast managers who were not of the same professional group were unrestrained by the profession's regulatory framework and believed that having the legitimacy to extend services in order to meet performance targets empowered staff.

The similarity between these outcomes and the recommendations of the *Enquiry into NHS Management (Griffiths Report)* (DHSS 1983) cannot be ignored. The report, undertaken by Roy Griffiths, then Deputy Chairman and Managing Director of Sainsburys, brought about the introduction of General Management to the NHS which had hitherto been 'administered' by Hospital Administrators. Others on the report team included senior management representation from other commercial organisations such as British Telecom and United Biscuits.

In essence the Griffiths Report concluded that within the NHS there was an absence of any coherent management at a local level and it lacked continuous evaluation of performance against any normal business criteria, which they identified as:

- Levels of service
- Quality of product
- Operating within budgets
- Cost improvement
- Productivity
- Motivating and rewarding staff
- Research and development.

Most significantly there was little evaluation of clinical practice and even less evaluation of the effectiveness of clinical interventions. Managers from industry, commerce and business were introduced by the end of 1985 and Clinical Directorates were established to lead on clinical management and excellence.

This relationship between practice and leadership is quite uniquely described by Maslow (1998) in his analogy between farming, successful crop production and the characteristics required for good leadership.

The good farmer simply throws out seeds, sets up good growing conditions and then gets out of the way....he doesn't pull up the growing seed to see if it's doing all right; the good leader is again like the farmer...not so much in forcing or shaping people but in offering them good growing conditions to grow without too much interference.

(Maslow, 1998, p.10)

The parallels between this description by Maslow and aspects of Storey's typology (Storey, 2004) are evident. Whilst management of situations may go beyond simply being desirable (it is at times essential), management through effective leadership which is enabling and empowering and something which transforms practice in a dynamic way rather than being a slave to policy and protocol and the 'tick box' approach to clinical governance, is more likely to yield better results and improve the morale of staff along the way.

Education Research and Clinical Management

Vernon and Campbell (2007) identify that the relationship of the profession to clinical management has been augmented significantly by the move in the mid-1990s, in the UK, to a graduate education, which took chiropodists beyond simply being trained to perform procedures but most importantly to create a research-based body of knowledge which came out of the profession itself.

Without research a professional group will not only be in danger of being seen as a second-class service but could also be seen to be unable to justify its own existence in terms of clinical effectiveness and could in turn become obsolete.

(Vernon & Campbell, 2007, p.3)

The significance of the historic absence of this body of knowledge can reasonably be argued to be an influencing factor as to why the profession occupied a period of stasis for several decades. It is clear that there have been significant developments within podiatric education, clinical practice and professional regulation (Ashford *et al.,* 1995; Kippen, 1995; Curran *et al.,* 2006; Institute for Innovation & Improvement, 2011; HPC, 2011). Good quality empirical research from within the profession will produce a body of knowledge which is podiatric in genesis and emphasis. This has the capacity to influence the clinical agenda and in turn to bolster and influence clinical management within podiatry. The need for such research has been recognised and steps to address this need are underway.

The observations made by Turlik *et al.* (2003), Porthouse and Torgerson (2004), Young (2007) and more recently by Hawke *et al.* (2009) regarding the dearth of reliable quantitative research were critical in different ways of the extent to which podiatric research is available in order to influence practice. This ranged from problems associated with ease of access to the research due to limited database resources which house and summarise the research through to lack of effective methods of disseminating the evidence within practice.

However the above data (see Figure 5.1) in relation to numbers of registered podiatrists in the UK, whilst certainly increasing, still show very clearly that as one of the smallest professional groups of Allied Health Professionals, they are likely to be the sole practitioner within multidisciplinary teams or if in private practice to function independently, autonomously and moreover without identifiable governance structures. This has potentially left podiatrists exposed, not only in terms of minimal colleague support or opportunity to work collaboratively with others in their specialism, but also in terms of the limited understanding of their expertise and scope of practice by others.

The issue of being a single handed practitioner, either as the sole podiatrist within statutory services' multidisciplinary teams or as a single-handed practitioner in private practice, is particularly highlighted by the Quality Assurance Agency for Higher Education (QAA) in a benchmarking statement for health professions courses (QAA, 2001). Here they identify curricular standards that the providing institution is expected to meet and the practice-based knowledge and competencies that students should be expected to attain in order to achieve their award and be deemed competent to practice. An understanding of the issues relating to professional practice and care of patients by sole practitioners within statutory services or commercial businesses is identified in several statements under the headings of professional and personal responsibilities.

Clinical Management and Podiatric Leadership

The management of clinical situations is commonplace in healthcare and no less so in podiatry (Harmonson & Harkless, 1996; Rijken *et al.*, 1999; Hawke *et al.*, 2009; Sanders *et al.*, 2010; Cockayne *et al.*, 2011; Leese *et al.*, 2011; Spink *et al.*, 2011). The use of clinical protocols, care pathways and standardised assessment processes across a range of specialities within healthcare provision are becoming equally commonplace (Mellor *et al.*, 2004; NICE 2005; Matthews *et al.*, 2006; Ahmad *et al.*, 2007; NICE 2010; Warren 2011; NICE 2011) but this leads us to consider the extent to which the input of podiatry has been recognised within care pathways and integrated care or the referral pathways of some chronic conditions. One example where the evidence is strongest is the (limited) provision of podiatric care within rheumatology services (Jacobi *et al.*, 2004; Redmond *et al.*, 2006; Taal *et al.*, 2006; Juarez *et al.*, 2010; Rome *et al.*, 2010) with significant variation in both quality and availability of services. Lack of knowledge or understanding regarding the need for good foot care for this patient group is generally not the issue. Whilst multidisciplinary input in relation to rheumatology care is also well established, what appears to be lacking is recognition of the need for effective and systematic podiatric care within rheumatology along the lines of that provided for patients with diabetes.

The perceived complexity of the clinical management required within healthcare specialities is argued to be influential in how and why professional recognition comes about. These arguments were expanded in the early 1980s by Skipper and Hughes (1983) and more recently by Mandy (2008) in exploring why podiatry had had difficulty in achieving ownership over and autonomy within its speciality.

One of the arguments has been that podiatry has remained a 'low status' profession because much of the clinical work relates to older populations.

> *Foot conditions worsen with age…the majority of patients in receipt of podiatric care are those over 50 years of age.*
>
> (Mandy, 2008, p. 202)

Conditions of the feet/lower legs are more prevalent in older populations either because of degenerative changes (Menz & Lord, 2005; Beeson *et al.*, 2009 & D'Arcangelo *et al.*, 2010, Juarez *et al.*, 2010) or because of comorbidities where podiatric care is considered an essential requirement. The consequences of foot related complications in diabetes can be catastrophic (Armstrong *et al.*, 1997; Lipsky *et al.*, 2006; Hunt, 2011; Margolis *et al.*, 2011; Mani *et al.*, 2011)

However Mandy (2008) also points out that with an ageing population the use of podiatric services, both for the perceived minor ailments and in utilising the extended scope of practice of podiatric surgery, may become more prevalent. In short demographic changes and the need to cater for a greater prevalence of chronic conditions which present with podiatric demands, such as diabetes, may open the door for greater utilisation of podiatry services. In fact the argument that podiatry should 'embrace' the demographics of its patient group and develop a speciality around elderly populations was put forward by Helfand (2000a; 2000b) with a proposal that podiatric medicine should pursue a Geriatric Fellowship in Podiatric Medicine, based upon postgraduate qualifications. This would encompass the responsibility to promote change, to be influential in care provision and in establishing policies and priorities in relation to foot care, in effect to exercise leadership within podiatry.

Leadership and Excellence in Podiatry

Skipper and Hughes (1995) made the observation that without doubt podiatric medical education has been greatly influenced by general medical education. The extent to which this influence can be further extended in order to enable podiatry to exercise clinical leadership and excellence in its own field is less clear. Alternatively the potential for podiatry to be recognised as able to offer leadership may come from its relationships closer to home, as an Allied Health Profession (AHP), with its nearest influencing professions being physiotherapy, occupational therapy, and drawing from the vast amount of literature which nursing has generated over the years.

The modernisation agenda within the NHS, established as part of the NHS Plan in 2000 (Department of Health (DOH), 2000) covered several aspects relating to access to services, waiting times, procurement and customer service, but no less important was the commitment regarding leadership across all occupational groups. Similarly in 2003:

> *...it will have fully developed leadership programmes for allied health professionals.* (Department of Health, 2003.)

The argument is that clinicians play a pivotal role in the delivery of clinical care and ought to be enabled to direct and influence change. This had been referred to earlier in the policy document, *Shifting the Balance of Power: The Next Steps* (DOH, 2002) which asserted that clinicians should be enabled to exercise greater decision making and, to facilitate this, clinical and professional leadership programmes would be established. Podiatry and chiropody are not mentioned specifically in the 2002 report and AHPs are referred to only once in the document, regarding securing leadership programmes:

> *The particular arrangements for this need to be determined locally with PCTs, NHS Trusts and StHAs all considering how they can secure good leadership of all the professions including the Allied Health Professions.* (DOH 2002, p. 16.)

It is difficult not to reach the conclusion that the Allied Health Professions are included as an afterthought, though whether this was the intention is impossible to assess. That AHPs are notable almost by their absence from the substance of this policy does raise the question as to the real commitment, at that time, to enabling leadership across all professional groups.

Consultant posts

Another development from the NHS modernisation agenda was to create consultant posts for nurses, midwives and allied health professionals. Research between 2007 and 2011 (Humphreys *et al.*, 2007; Humphreys *et al.*, 2010, Stevenson, 2011) has attempted to evaluate this role but on looking in detail at the studies undertaken (Humphreys *et al.*, 2007, 2010) the actual involvement of AHPs, let alone podiatry, is minimal and the inclusion of studies in the 2007 paper is much wider than the title of the paper would suggest. The focus is not only on the role of the nurse/allied health consultant but includes a great many studies where some aspect of what might be covered in the role of the consultant is evaluated, but not necessarily in people who were employed in consultant posts.

The criteria evaluated are those regarded as the four pillars of the consultant post:

- expert practice
- leadership

- education
- research.

The 2007 study did not identify any AHP consultants, although it did identify AHP practitioners encompassing some of the four pillars in their role. Neither podiatry/podiatrist, chiropody/chiropodist were included in the systematic search criteria; the 2010 study sampled five Nurse Consultants and one Physiotherapy Consultant. In Stevenson (2011) the sample of seven consultants comprised five nurses, one physiotherapist and one pharmacist. The evidence tells us that whilst there have been minor gains made in the consultant posts occupied by some AHPs, podiatry was absent from any of these studies and the continued evidence is that nursing and midwifery continue to occupy the majority of the non-medical consultant roles as defined by and established from the NHS Plan (DOH, 2000).

Leadership styles

Leadership styles and characteristics are heavily influential in whether the endeavours to bring about change are successful or not and also in what makes for successful leadership (Kotter,1995; Fiol *et al.*, 1999; Bommer *et al.*, 2005; Mrkonjic & Grondin, 2011). Some of the significant aspects regarding the debate on leadership have been presented in a recent overview (Hartley & Benington, 2010) and in particular some of the ambiguity relating to what exactly is leadership. Hitherto within healthcare, leadership has been located with the seniority of positions, the organisational structure and reflected in rewards, remuneration, pay and conditions. However if taken at its simplest, leadership is argued to be:

> *...the process of influencing people in the formulation of or pursuit of goals then potentially everyone working in healthcare can be a leader, at sometime for some purpose.*   (Hartley & Benington, 2010 p.26.)

If this is accepted as both reasonable and achievable then the concept of leadership within healthcare inverts; it becomes something more akin to democracy than hierarchy, position and authority. Rather than it being viewed as a responsibility invested in a few to lead the many, it becomes a more radical proposal whereby everyone can be empowered to lead rather than simply be led. It is difficult to imagine that this is what was intended within the *Griffiths Report* (DHSS, 1983), *The*

NHS Plan (DOH, 2000) or *Shifting the Balance of Power: the Next Steps* (DOH, 2002) in that these policy documents aimed to create organisational change and produce organisational structures where leadership would happen and where leaders would be located.

The Clinical Leadership Competency Framework Project (2010)

More recently however the findings of the Clinical Leadership Competency Framework Project (Institute for Innovation and Improvement, 2011) identify the state of readiness in the UK for embedding leadership within education and training for all professions and occupational groups registered with the HPC, nurses (and health visitors), midwives and social workers. Podiatry occupies a place in this by virtue of its statutory regulator being the HPC. Addressing the issue of leadership for these professional groups comes from 'rolling the process back' so that leadership as a professional requisite is an essential component of pre-registration education and training rather than something which only becomes a feature of senior post job descriptions and role specifications.

The HPC is argued to be key in being able to influence the introduction of a Clinical Leadership Competency Framework (CLCF) within the current pre-registration education arena; in order to be registered as an HPC practitioner an honours degree in podiatry is necessary. As a professional body the Society of Chiropodists and Podiatrists is in a position to include leadership within post-registration education, although at present there is no compulsory Continuing Professional Development (CPD) requirement which specifically covers leadership.

Given that the CLCF venture is in its infancy, with consultation having taken place only in 2010, it is impossible to say what a picture of success might look like or how the vision of embedding leadership into podiatry education and thus practice will be realised. If leadership is to be emancipatory and widespread within AHP and podiatry, in the way that Hartley and Benington (2010) argue it could be, then the CLCF might be in a position to make this happen by ensuring leadership becomes everyone's business. It could then be an essential part of podiatry education and practice and not just limited to high earning, high esteem posts or wheeled out when service re-design is necessary or when inspirational leaders are required to bring about the next round of structural changes necessary to keep health services afloat in an ever changing health economy.

Conclusion

The emergence of management and leadership within podiatry has been something of a difficult birth. The history surrounding education, training, recruitment, retention and statutory regulation along with the perceived low status of the profession and limitations in good quality empirical research produced by podiatrists have made for something of a difficult journey. However it is clear that in the UK since 2004 many of these obstacles and deficiencies are being addressed. In the years 2003 to 2011, for the first time since the mid-1960s, the percentage increase of registered podiatrists exceeded that of other comparable professions registered with the HPC, with numbers of podiatrists registered with the HPC increasing from just over 9,000 in 2003 to in excess of 12,700 in November 2011. Previously it had taken 37 years for podiatry numbers to rise from their baseline figure of 4,530 in 1967 to 9013 in 2003 (HPC, 2011).

The comparative literature regarding management and leadership, both generically and as applied to podiatry presents a varied landscape. Whilst the literature allows for both comparison and contrast of management and leadership it is also clear that applying business and commercial qualities to healthcare has not been without its difficulties. The recent interpretation of leadership as being something which everyone is both capable of and should engage in as a professional obligation has changed the landscape once again. Leadership, as a competency to be fulfilled within education and practice, which can and ought to be expected of all practitioners, rather than the preserve of those who come to sort out services, teams and departments when it goes wrong, is without doubt a radical change from the traditional view that there are inspirational leaders and there are the rest, those who are led. The extent to which this revised view of leadership and leaders will do what is envisaged remains to be seen. What is clear is that health economics will continue to influence the development of podiatry education and practice in the future, just as it has done in the past.

References

Ahmad, F., Roy, A., Brady, S., Belgeonne, S., Dunn, L. and Pitts, J. (2007). 'Care pathway initiative for people with intellectual disabilities: impact evaluation' in *Journal of Nursing Management*, **15**(7): 700–702.

Armstrong, D.G., Lavery, L.A., Quebedeaux, T.L. and Walker, S.C. (1997). 'Surgical morbidity and the risk of amputation due to infected puncture wounds in diabetic versus nondiabetic adults' in *Journal of the American Podiatric Medical Association*, **87**(7): 321–326.

Ashford, R.L., Tollafield, D.R. and Axe, D. (1995). 'Podiatry education in the UK' in *The Foot*, **5**(1): 1–7.

Beeson, P., Phillips, C., Corr, S. and Ribbans, W. (2009). 'Hallux rigidus: a cross-sectional study to evaluate clinical parameters' in *The Foot*, **19**(2): 80–92.

Blakeman, P.D. (2003). 'Management styles and professional identities among UK podiatrists' in *The International Journal of Public Sector Management,* **16** (2): 131–140.

Bommer,W.H., Rich, G.A. and Rubin, R.S. (2005). 'Changing attitudes about change: Longitudinal effects of transformational leader behavior on employee cynicism about organizational change' in *Journal of Organizational Behavior*, **26**(7): 733–753.

Cockayne, S., Curran, M., Denby, G., Hashmi, F., Hewitt, C., Hicks, K., Jayakody, S., Kangombe, A., McIntosh, C. and McLarnon, N. (2011). 'EVerT: cryotherapy versus salicylic acid for the treatment of verrucae – a randomised controlled trial' in *Health Technology Assessment*, **15**(32): 1–17.

Curran, M.J., Campbell, J. and Rugg, G. (2006). 'An investigation into the clinical reasoning of both expert and novice podiatrists' in *The Foot*, **16**(1): 28–32.

D'Arcangelo, P.R., Landorf, K.B., Munteanu, S.E., Zammit, G.V. and Menz, H.B. (2010). 'Radiographic correlates of hallux valgus severity in older people' in *Journal of Foot and Ankle Research*, (3): 20.

Department of Health & Social Services (1983). *Enquiry into NHS Managment, (Griffiths Report)*, London: HMSO.

Department of Health (2000). *The NHS Plan: a plan for investment, a plan for reform*. London: HMSO.

Department of Health (2002). *Shifting the Balance of Power: The Next Steps*. London: HMSO. Available at: www.dh.gov.uk/en/Publicationsandstatistics/Publications/PublicationsPolicyAndGuidance/DH_4002960 (accessed 19/06/12).

Department of Health (2003). *The NHS Plan – a progress report. (The NHS Modernisation Board Annual Report 2003)*. London: HMSO.

Drucker, P. (1993). *Post-capitalist Society*. New York: Harper Collins.

Fiol, C.M., Harris, D. and House, R. (1999). 'Charismatic leadership: Strategies for effecting social change' in *Leadership Quarterly*, **10**(3): 449–482.

Harmonson, J.K. and Harkless, L.B. (1996). 'Operative procedures for the correction of hammertoe, claw toe, and mallet toe: a literature review' in *Clinical Podiatric Medicine and Surgery*, April; **13**(2): 211–220.

Hartley, J. and Benington, J. (2010). *Leadership for Healthcare*. Bristol, UK: The Policy Press.

Hawke, F., Burns, J. and Landorf, K.B. (2009). 'Evidence-based podiatric medicine: importance of systematic reviews in clinical practice' in *Journal of the American Podiatric Medical Association*, **99**(3): 260–266.

Health Professions Council (2011) Current Statistics.
Available at: http://www.hpcuk.org/aboutregistration/theregister/stats/ (accessed 16/06/12)

Helfand, A.E. (2000a). 'A conceptual model for a geriatric syllabus for podiatric medicine' in *Journal of the American Podiatric Medical Association*, May; 90(5): 258–267.

Helfand, A.E. (2000b). 'A conceptual model for a geriatric fellowship in podiatric medicine' in *Journal of the Amercian Podiatric Medical Association*, June; **90**(6): 313–319.

Humphreys, A., Johnson, S., Richardson, J. Stenhouse, E. and Watkins, M. (2007). 'Systematic review and meta-synthesis: evaluating the effectiveness of nurse, midwife and allied health professional consultants' in *Journal of Clinical Nursing*, **16**(10): 1792–1808.

Humphreys, A., Richardson, J., Stenhouse, E. and Watkins, E. (2010). 'Assessing the impact of nurse and allied health professional consultants: developing an activity diary' in *Journal of Clinical Nursing*, **19** (17–18): 2565–2573.

Hunt, D.L. (2011). 'Diabetes: foot ulcers and amputations' in *Clinical Evidence* (Online) Aug 26 pii: 0602.

Institute for Innovation & Improvement (2011). *Clinical Leadership Competency Framework Project.*
Available at: http://www.institute.nhs.uk/building_capability/building_leadership_capability/clinical_leadership_competency_framework_project.html (accessed 16/06/12).

Jacobi, C.E., Triemstra, M., Rupp, I. Dinant, H.J. and Van Den Bas, G.A. (2001). 'Health care utilization among rheumatoid arthritis patients referred to a rheumatology center: unequal needs, unequal care?' in *Arthritis and Rheumatism,* **45**(4): 324–330.

Juarez, M., Price, E., Collins, D. and Williamson, L. (2010). 'Deficiencies in provision of integrated multidisciplinary podiatry care for patients with inflammatory arthritis: A UK district general hospital experience' in *The Foot,* (20): 71–74.

Kippen, C. (1995). 'Podiatry education in New Zealand' in *The Foot,* (4): 167–169.

Kotter, J. (1990). *What Leaders Really Do.* Boston, MA: Harvard Business School Press.

Kotter, J. (1995). 'Leading change: Why transformation efforts fail' in *Harvard Business Review,* **73**(2): 59–67.

Leese, G.P., Cochrane, L., Mackie, A.D., Strong, D., Brown, K. and Green, V. (2011). 'Measuring the accuracy of different ways to identify the "at-risk" foot in routine clinical practice' in *Diabetic Medicine,* **28**(6): 747–754.

Lipsky, B.A., Berendt, A.R., Deery, H.G., Embil, J.M., Joseph, W.S., Karchmer, A.W., LeFrock, J.L., Lew, D.P., Mader, J.T., Norden, C. and Tan, J.S. (2006). 'Treatment of Diabetic Foot Infections' in *Plastic and Reconstructive Surgery,* **117**; 7 [Suppl]: 212S–238S.

Mandy, P. (2008). 'The status of podiatry in the United Kingdom' in *The Foot,* **18**: 202–205.

Mani, R., Yarde, S. and Edmonds, M. (2011). 'Prevalence of deep venous incompetence and microvascular abnormalities in patients with diabetes mellitus' in *The International Journal of Lower Extremity Wounds,* **10**(2): 75–79.

Margolis, D.J., Hoffstad, O., Nafash, J., Leonard, C.E., Freeman, C.P., Hennessy, S. and Weibe, D.J. (2011). 'Location, location, location: geographic clustering of lower-extremity amputation among medicare beneficiaries with diabetes' in *Diabetes Care,* **34**(11): 2363–2367.

Maslow, A. (1998). *Maslow on Management.* New York: John Wiley & Sons Inc.

Matthews, K., Gambles, M., Ellershaw, J.E., Brook, L., Williams, M., Hodgson, A. and Barber, M. (2006). 'Developing the Liverpool Care Pathway for the dying child' in *Paediatric Nursing* **18**(1): 18–21.

Mellor, F., Foley, T., Connolly, M., Mercer, V. and Spanswick, M. (2004). 'Role of a clinical facilitator in introducing an integrated care pathway for the care of the dying' in *International Journal of Palliative Nursing,* **10**(10): 497–501.

Menz, H.B. and Lord, S.R. (2005). 'Gait instability in older people with hallux valgus' in *Foot and Ankle International,* **26**(6):483–489.

Mrkonjic, L. and Grondin, S.C. (2011). 'Introduction to concepts in leadership for the surgeon' *Thoracic Surgery Clinics,* **21**(3): 323–331.

NICE (2005). The recognition and initial management of ovarian cancer.
Available at: http://www.nice.org.uk/nicemedia/live/13464/54194/54194.pdf (accessed 17/06/12).

NICE (2010). Reducing differences in the uptake of immunisations (PH21).
Available at: www.nice.org.uk/PH21 (accessed 17/06/12).

NICE (2011). Surgical correction of hallux valgus using minimal access techniques.
Available at: guidance.nice.org.uk/IPG332 (accessed 19/06/12).

Nursing & Midwifery Council (2011). *Nursing and Midwifery Council: Annual Fitness to Practice Report 2010-2011*. London: NMC.

Porthouse, J. and Torgerson, D.J. (2004). 'The need for randomized controlled trials in podiatric medical research' in *Journal of the American Podiatric Medical Association*, **94**(3): 221–228.

The Quality Assurance Agency for Higher Education (2001). *Benchmark Statement: Health care programmes. Phase 1*. Gloucester: QAA.

Redmond, A.C., Waxman, R. and Helliwell, P.S. (2006). 'Provision of foot health services in rheumatology in the UK' in *Rheumatology*, **45**(5): 571–576.

Rijken, P.M., Dekker, J., Lankhorst, G.J., Dekker, E., Bakker, K., Dooren, J. and Rauwerda, J.A.(1999). 'Podiatric care for diabetic patients with foot problems: an observational study' in *International Journal of Rehabilitation Research*, **22**(3): 181–188.

Rome, K., Chapman, J., Williams, A.E., Gow, P. and Dalbeth, N. (2010). 'Podiatry services for patients with arthritis: an unmet need' in *New Zealand Medical Journal*, **123**(1310): 91-97.

Rousseau, J.J. (1972). *On Education*. New York: Dutton.

Sanders, L.J., Robbins, J.M. and Edmonds, M.E. (2010). 'History of the team approach to amputation prevention: pioneers and milestones' in *Journal of the American Podiatric Medical Association*, **100**(5): 317–34.

Skipper, J.K. and Hughes, J.E. (1983). 'Podiatry: A medical care specialty in quest of full professional status and recognition' in *Social Science & Medicine* **17**:(20) 1541–1548.

Skipper, J. and Hughes, J. (1995). 'Podiatry: a medical care speciality in quest of full professional status and recognition' in *Readings in American Health Care: Current Issues In Socio-Historical Perspective*, W.G. Rothstein (ed). Madison, WI: The University of Wisconsin Press.

Spink, M.J., Fotoohabadi, M.R. and Wee, E. (2011). 'Predictors of adherence to a multifaceted podiatry intervention for the prevention of falls in older people' in *BioMed Central Geriatrics*, **11**(51) 1–8.

Stevenson, K., Ryan, S. and Masterson, A. (2011). 'Nurse and allied health professional consultants: perceptions and experiences of the role' in *Journal of Clinical Nursing*, **20**(3–4): 537–544.

Storey, J. (2004). *Leadership in Organisations*. Abingdon: Routledge.

Taal, E., Bobietinska, E., Lloyd, J. Veehof, M., Rasker, W.J., Oosterveld, F.G. and Rasker, J.J. (2006). 'Successfully living with chronic arthritis. The role of the allied health professionals' in *Clinical Rheumatology*, **25**(2): 189–197.

Turlik, M.A., Kushner, D. and Stock, D. (2003). 'Assessing the validity of published randomized controlled trials in podiatric medical journals' in *Journal of the American Podiatric Medical Association*, **93**(5): 392–398.

Vernon, W. and Campbell, J. (2007). 'The why, who and what of podiatry research' in *A Guide to Research for Podiatrists*, J.Campbell (ed.). Keswick: M&K Update Ltd.

Warren, D. (2011). 'Implementation of a protocol for the prevention and management of extravasation injuries in the neonatal intensive care patient' in *International Journal of Evidence-Based Healthcare* **9**(2): 165–171.

Young, G. (2007). 'Evidence-based medicine in podiatric residency training' in *Clinical Podiatric Medicine and Surgery*, **24**(1): 11–6

Yukl, G.A. (2006). *Leadership in Organizations* (6th edn). Englewood Cliffs, NJ: Prentice-Hall.

Chapter Six

Building Strategic Curricula in Podiatric Medicine

Dr Catherine Hayes

Setting the Scene for Podiatric Curriculum Development

Enabling students to acquire the knowledge and skills which will allow them to make a lasting difference to society, not just the healthcare arena is now a fundamental priority for curriculum development in podiatric medicine. How and what students learn along with what is actually being taught is pivotal; due consideration of what we are equipping practitioners for and in laying groundwork for an integrated development of the education of a globally employed podiatric practitioner workforce is now a necessity.

Within the context of podiatric education, the majority of curriculum design for programmes, whether undergraduate or postgraduate, has stemmed from assumptions that learning is a one-dimensional concept with definitive starting and completion points, undertaken by the individual student in pursuit of knowledge. This knowledge is perceived both as being consumed by the learner and requiring a formalised process of teaching in order to separate it from the rest of everyday activity and experience. Traditional assertions such as these are fundamentally flawed, yet the theories proposed by Lave and Wenger as far back as the 1980s and 1990s have still failed to provide a panacea for academic curriculum development which truly addresses the complexities posed by multidisciplinary and interdisciplinary learning (Kerno, 2008). Historically, the most significant of these theories was 'Situated Learning', which focuses on learning within a 'Community of Practice' and addresses the social dimension of learning as a core activity of human existence. This original approach can be effectively adapted for a more innovative approach to curriculum design and justification (Lave and Wenger, 1991). Whilst this educational model offers no greater panacea for the challenges of a strategically designed curriculum, what it does offer is the opportunity to individualise and tailor teaching and learning for a diverse array of podiatry students, incorporating the core features of social and cultural competency (Eaton *et al.*, 2011).

Rationalising a Different Approach

The rationale for adopting a development of Lave and Wenger's Situated Learning (SL) within podiatric curriculum development is relatively straightforward; a strategic workforce needs to be equipped with practitioners whose core clinical proficiency is underpinned by a clear ability to make informed decisions on the best evidence available.

This chapter presents the case for merging the theoretical underpinnings of SL with the concept of Problem Based Learning (PBL), in which knowledge is created rather than consumed. This involves a different approach to curriculum design and implementation, which is responsive to the need to build capacity within and between professional disciplines across the healthcare arena.

The prospect of deconstructing years of traditional educational provision is one which challenges the whole certainty of academic curriculum design and the mechanisms of teaching, learning and assessment which are a fundamental and integral part of it.

> Adopting a combination of Situated Learning and Problem Based Learning offers one innovative mechanism of educational provision for podiatric practitioners with students learning together in a community of practice driven by curriculum content. The aim of this approach is to facilitate the acquisition of a highly developed and transferable skill base in lower limb assessment, diagnosis and management, relevant to the needs of patients.

The merging of these two educational theories is one means by which podiatric curriculum development might evolve. In the long term it represents a mechanism whereby academic curricula can be essentially future proofed in terms of their capacity to provide what healthcare organisations actually need rather than what Higher Education Institutes think they need. Perhaps more significantly how providers of education might deliver a proactive and highly quantifiable response can be addressed in a practically feasible and educationally rigorous approach.

Curriculum development is fundamental if podiatry is to become a leading allied healthcare profession and attain the formal recognition that has hitherto eluded it.

Philosophical Underpinnings of a New Approach to Curriculum Development

Within the field of education, basic sociocultural perspectives on the acquisition of knowledge and process of learning originated from critical commentaries of Dewey's philosophical base of pragmatism (Westbrook, 2005), seminal work on the concept of social constructivism (Piaget, 1950), Vygotsky's cultural historical theory (Liu and Matthews, 2005) and Bakhtin's dialogism (Brandist, 2002). Whilst Piaget, focused heavily on the metacognitive processes of the learner, in contrast, the socioculturally oriented theoretical approaches to constructivism regarded the construction of knowledge as essentially social and embedded in a community of practitioners (Wenger, 1998).

Within the context of learning, regardless of level, it is the dimensional approaches to learning described by Vygotsky which are theoretically significant to the process of curriculum development in podiatric medicine. The interrelationship of different levels of learning is significant since it allows examination of the role of human development within peer groups, in particular the impact of human discourse and dialogue on the nature and type of learning (Cornelissen *et al.*, 2011). In addition to this, activity theory can be used as a mechanism of linking learning to the broader reality, that is, how tacit knowledge might be applied in the real world of clinical professional practice (Daniels, 2008).

In terms of strategic curriculum development, an examination of sociocultural theory warrants a clear focus on the nature and context of knowledge and an acknowledgement of:

- the situated nature of knowledge
- the social origin and impact of knowledge
- the distribution of knowledge
- the mediation of knowledge
- the dependence of knowledge acquisition upon language and discourse
- the dependence upon human intrinsic motivation to ensure participation in the active process of learning
- the nature of communities of practice needed for knowledge to be real not rhetoric.

Individually Tailoring a Model of Curricula for Health

The educational theory of SL which could potentially underpin future podiatric curricula is one which differs distinctly from traditional didactic approaches to teaching and learning in higher education, and is more suited to the professional practice requirements of people engaging in vocational as well as academic study. The concept of role development and the acquisition of clearly focused and well rationalised clinical knowledge and skills is paramount. Programmes should also be designed to acknowledge the impact of studying on life as a whole and not merely as an academic exercise, to accommodate the diversity of students' circumstances. As a direct result of the strategic and holistic design of podiatric curricula, students should be better equipped to manage their studies alongside the demands of everyday life.

Curricula in healthcare reflect the need for the practical application of cognate knowledge to the environment of working with patients at the front line of care (Jovchelovitch, 2007). This necessitates a holistic approach to curriculum design and implementation. The creation rather than the consumption of knowledge is the premise of this approach, which promotes an active engagement of the podiatry student with the process of learning and how best their own motivation to learn can ultimately drive mechanisms of assessment and achievement (Anderson & Krathwohl, 2001). Where some curricula fall short is in the failure of their initial design and a lack of recognition that true learning captures the essence of a person's being and is not merely a process of knowledge acquisition. The fundamental characteristics of successful educational curricula (Krathwohl *et al.*, 1964) can be outlined as follows:

- an unambiguous approach to the explanation of learning aims and objectives.
- a research based and theory driven approach
- establishing a community of practice
- building core transferability of generic skill
- personalising the learning experience for individual motivation
- compounding the opportunity for the building of core competence
- ensuring the applied functionality of knowledge
- progressive assessment of stages of learning development
- embedding of social learning into the curriculum
- provision of networking opportunities beyond programme context
- a clear focus on cultural inclusivity
- addressing the notion of continuing professional development.

The longstanding debate as to whether knowledge acquisition in the context of higher education actually translates into the effective application of knowledge in practice at the front line of patient care continues (Matthews *et al.*, 2011). In order to address this in the strategic development of podiatric curricula the central tenets of **knowledge contextualisation**, **framing** and **constructing** must be addressed (Levinson & Pizzo, 2011). The creation of knowledge in the context of application to practice has been the fundamental basis of teaching and learning within podiatric medicine for decades. Perhaps the unique engagement and interaction we share with our patient caseloads can be argued as one of the main drivers for the creation of new knowledge and its application to practice. One neglected area within the context of this mechanism of education is how students can be equipped with the degree of generic skill transferability from the context of an educational programme to the context of the workplace (Raymond-Seniuk & Profetto-McGrath, 2011).

The Difference with a Problem Based Learning Approach

Conventional curricula in podiatric medicine delivered by traditional didactic educational practices cover individual subjects of study which are often only applicable to the specific professional disciplines within which we work. Where we are privileged in the field of podiatric medicine is in the broad spread of subject disciplines being taught, none of which are completely specific to the profession and none of which could not be undertaken by other healthcare professionals. This places podiatrists as potential keystones in the foundation for building capacity within and between professional healthcare disciplines since our integration is founded not only on an understanding of core subjects in health and medicine but an active engagement in them. By using the advocated 'PBL Approach' in conjunction with this philosophical ethos we can fundamentally equip students with the ability to engage with core knowledge understanding and values as well as the capacity to engage and interact with other professions within the context of patient centred care (Lown *et al.*, 2011). What is necessary however is the fundamental need for an institutional approach to the implementation of PBL in practice across the whole academic curriculum and not just sparse parts of it. Through this it is then possible to begin to change not just a culture of learning but also the culture of its facilitation and the future shaping of a dynamic and responsive profession.

The Challenge of Developing Assessment Mechanisms

One of the greatest challenges with this technique of knowledge acquisition and creation is in the choice of assessment adopted within the curriculum and how these processes and mechanisms can be effectively implemented across the major domains of learning (Neville, 2009). Where core failure in this process has the potential to occur is in the use of traditional didactic assessment mechanisms which cannot drive the intrinsic processes of teaching and learning which will build the individual motivation to succeed directly into podiatric curricula.

The mechanism of assessment of programmes should be specifically designed to assess the level of performance of students in the articulation of their ideas and strategies within the context of clinical professional practice to provide a tacit and real demonstration of their engagement and application of the programme content to real life practice (Colbert *et al.*, 2009).

In the 'PBL approach', which integrates the concept of SL with PBL, students should begin with relevant clinical problems and with the help of a facilitator work out how much they effectively do know and understand of the core knowledge they already have and subsequently that which they do not know. They should then actively be able to define what they need to learn in order to fully understand the problems they encounter in everyday clinical and professional practice. What students study is therefore more clearly defined by the needs of their own individual and situated context of professional practice as well as being determined by a robust series of learning opportunities within the cognate disciplines of science which underpin the practice of podiatric medicine.

Short case scenarios (cases) should be used to start and guide the process of learning at both undergraduate and postgraduate levels. Emphasis should be placed on the gaps that students discover in their knowledge and skills, and how to bridge these gaps with new knowledge, understanding and behaviour patterns. In this respect the PBL approach will aim to enable students to discover and learn for themselves, facilitated by experienced tutors. This system replaces traditional didactic teaching methods and enables learning, through the creation of a cohesive learning group.

The Significance of PBL Problems

In a curriculum adopting a PBL approach, the choice of problems is hugely significant. The choices and the framework within which they should be presented should be determined by three main criteria:

- Key issues of knowledge underpinning clinical practice in the general context of health and wellbeing in healthcare.
- Key concepts in hands on clinical practice fundamental to overall improved patient assessment, diagnosis and management.
- Key concepts in the holistic development of practitioners and how their societal as well as professional contribution can be enhanced through a rigorous education process.

In embedding processes of education within problems which bring to life the practical application of knowledge in the context of patient-centred care, students should then be afforded the opportunity of assessing in a risk-free environment the potential impact of applying their newly acquired knowledge to clinical practice. This also allows for the purposeful use of resources across various stages of the curriculum without the need for the active reinvention of materials (Juliano *et al.*, 2010).

Each element of new curricula should consist of a series of clinically related problems, which students use to define their specific study objectives in subjects from across the curriculum on a day-by-day basis. Students should work collaboratively in developing a firm understanding of aspects of podiatric medicine fundamental to either their foundation level studies in the profession at undergraduate level or alternatively at postgraduate level within their own branch of clinical professional practice.

Broader Issues of Curriculum Design and Development

All podiatric curricula should be designed to embed wider skills of knowledge and critical thinking and clinical leadership across their academic content in order to equip practitioners with the practical skills necessary for the management of the fundamental components of the wider public health agenda in the context of clinical professional practice (Dharamsi *et al.*, 2011). The generic skill base students acquire should be taught and facilitated by an array of subject experts with extensive experience of clinical practice in the context of healthcare organisations in primary and secondary healthcare settings. It should be expected that all students will contribute fully to interactive workshop and teaching sessions where PBL scenarios from an array of interprofessional and multi-disciplinary contexts are used. The aim is to form, develop and extend clinical practitioner knowledge in the field of clinical podiatric practice through the pivotal concept of patient-centred care (Cunningham *et al.*, 2011).

Active Learning Can Drive Purposeful Mechanisms of Assessment

The fundamental basis of podiatric curricula should be to enable qualified practitioners to perform a strategic and needs-led role both within the teams of which they are an integral part and within the broader context of capacity building between professional disciplines for the ultimate benefit of the patient (Rodriguez *et al.*, 2008). The active learning which is an integral feature of such a model would be destroyed by traditionally didactic mechanisms of prescriptive assessment. Developing programmes of study which allow a conglomerate group of healthcare practitioners to live and work together within the context of Continuing Professional Development (CPD) is a challenge. This also raises the possibility of a move beyond homogenous and bland lists of assessment criteria. Attention should therefore be shifted from the processes of assessment to its outcomes, which will ultimately translate rhetoric into reality upon successful execution of the curriculum (Ponsky, 2004).

Best Practice in Facilitation

Through a set of generic learning outcomes, students should be facilitated in their individual choice of how exactly they will fulfil them. This should be constructively aligned with the domain and nature of the learning they wish to submit as their evidence for reaching the intended learning outcomes. The evidence submitted will be as individual as every individual student on the programme. The use of portfolios as a mechanism of showcasing learning in practice should become a fundamental feature of most podiatric curricula, with emphasis on the need for educational mentorship through the process of submission rather than purely instructive direction on their format (Webb, 2009). Depending upon these specific domains of learning there are various examples of what students might wish to incorporate into their assignments across the curricula. Each domain of learning can then be individually assessed using specifically designed rubrics, which are in turn constructively aligned.

Research evidence demonstrates that one of the aspects of learning which students value highly is the ability to engage socially with those with whom they learn and those with whom they share a common experience or domain. This approach to learning also promotes the concept of **critical reflexivity** rather than a one-dimensional approach to reflective practice traditionally adopted within academic health curricula. This approach was originally termed 'situated learning' by Lave and Wenger in 1991 and has evolved in recent years to encompass how positive learning experiences are closely linked to the processes of regular human interaction with fellow students for whom learning is a shared endeavour and also the staff involved in clinical placement opportunities (Williamson *et al.*, 2011). Wenger's extension of the Theory of Situated Learning was further developed in 2008 by Kerno to provide a clear definitive terminology of what exactly differentiates a community of practice from other traditional cohorts of learners and also potential limitations to the approach (Kerno, 2008).

Wenger emphasised three definitive characteristics of a community of practice, namely:

Community: This term hinges on the notion that since students are brought together collectively to pursue their motivation to engage in teaching and learning in a particular domain, they are much more likely to be capable of engagement in group discussions, sharing information, the ability to socially support one another within a programme of study and the creation of lasting social relationships which add value to life beyond the confines of a learning environment and may well extend into leisure activity.

Domain: A community of practice is dependent upon a shared commitment to achieving a common goal. This shared commitment to achieving within a podiatric medicine curriculum should clearly differentiate this group of students from others who may be engaging in more traditional didactic pathways of academic study.

Practice: Podiatric medicine students are practitioners who share sustained experiences of social interaction through a period dedicated to shared educational/ clinical resources, shared narratives or stories, mechanisms of addressing the challenges of healthcare practice over the forthcoming years.

Contextualising and Framing Knowledge

Through these processes, instead of positioning tacit knowledge carefully within a traditional academic curriculum it will be allowed to emerge through participation in a framework specifically engineered to facilitate social learning. Social learning spaces are thus imperative to the success of programmes adopting this model of curriculum development.

Another part of the rationale for adopting this approach is the potential positive impact that this curriculum innovation might have upon recruitment and retention rates for which the impact of social support mechanisms cannot be underestimated; particularly within the context of undergraduate curricula. Defining clearly the needs of individual learning also fits with the ethos of this approach to applied pedagogy. Where the learning needs of student cohorts are accommodated, it is anticipated that students are better equipped to cope with their chosen designated learning outcomes with a remarkable individual impact upon clinical practice and social interaction with patients due to their own greater degree of self awareness (Symons *et al.*, 2009).

The Perry assumption, that all learners progress through a personal journey which encompasses intellectual and moral developments, is useful in progressively mapping individual opportunities for students to grow both professionally and personally (Perry, 1970). This is a particularly significant issue when we consider the ever changing dynamics of students' backgrounds and what they have already experienced in terms of their career pathways to date, if anything and also how this educational experience will become an embedded and integral part of their overall life experience (Perry, 1981).

Models and Theories of Cognitive Development and Progression

Broadly speaking these can be categorised as:

A. The Concept of Dualism and the Acquisition of Knowledge:

This deals specifically with the fact that there are definitively right and wrong answers which are indisputable. This in itself incorporates the fundamental concepts of:

Foundational or Basic Duality
This makes the assumption that all problems are solvable and therefore emphasis for the student has to be placed on actually learning the correct solutions to these problems with little room to manoeuvre.

Full Dualism
This refers to the fact that not all knowledge is absolute and that in some disciplines such as philosophy there can be no absolute correct answers, whereas in subjects of a more purist discipline there are right answers with no room for deviance or debate, for example within the sphere of mathematics or chemistry.

B. The Concept of Multiplicitous or Subjective Knowledge

This acknowledges the concept of there being conflicting answers, which may be based on experiential learning and experience of podiatrists within practice. This has often been referred to as anecdotal evidence and in terms of a hierarchy of evidence ranks poorly. However this can be further subdivided into:

Early Multiplicity:
Broadly categorised into problems in which:

- solutions are known and established and
- solutions which are not yet known and subsequently not yet established.

These concepts are then embedded together and in a process of dualism the podiatry student is actively facilitated in learning how to find a right solution.

Late Multiplicity:
Within the context of podiatric medicine, and working with people, which are essentially unquantifiable then the vast majority of problems are of the second type, which then leads to either of the two assumptions that:

a) Everyone has a right to their own opinion.
b) Some problems are essentially not solvable and therefore the relative solutions posed are irrelevant.

Interestingly, the tendencies of students choosing to study podiatric curricula are predictably drawn to the latter whereby human interaction is at the centre of the vast majority of their learning.

C. The Concept of Relative or Procedural Knowledge

This draws on the concept of there being disciplinary methods of reasoning based on the concepts of connected knowledge, which hinge on past experiential learning, and separated knowledge, which involves the active deconstruction of a presenting problem so that any pre-learned techniques for development can be adopted to begin resolving focal issues.

D. Contextual Relativism

This brackets off the assumption that all proposed solutions are underpinned by a solid rationale and that they can only be examined in context and rationalised by relative evidence. This gives a value to the 'situatedness' of learning and the focus for the podiatry student then becomes the development of the ability to evaluate the quality of solutions.

Prior Commitment and the Intrinsic Motivation to Engage

This hinges upon the ability of podiatric medicine students to engage with the necessity to:

- make informed choices;
- commit to valid and practically applicable solutions.

E. Integration of Constructed Knowledge into a Permanent Part of Being

Integration of knowledge learned from others with personal experience and reflection.

Actual Commitment

Student makes an actual commitment to the knowledge they have gained in order to apply it to practice.

Challenges to Commitment of Knowledge

In this context, the student will experience the implications of having their committed knowledge challenged where the student explores their own individual issues of responsibility.

Post-Commitment Acknowledgement

The student subsequently acknowledges that a commitment to knowledge within the context of learning can only be an ongoing and integral part of their role in clinical professional practice.

Within this process students can repeat their journey throughout the course of their career pathway and different domains of learning can often be at different stages at the same time. This has the ultimate and beneficial impact of:

- future proofing academic provision at both undergraduate and postgraduate level by establishing a unique and fundamental system of embedded responses to the need to change within healthcare delivery and practice;
- providing a fundamental basis for the proposed future provision of modern high quality, cohesively delivered curricula accredited, where appropriate, by our professional body;
- allowing the consideration and implementation of new innovative approaches to curriculum design and implementation in the real world.

Conclusion

In terms of improving approaches to curriculum development in podiatric medicine there are several additional factors which can further focus our unique contribution to the healthcare arena. If we actively allow assessment processes to drive teaching and learning through engagement of students in teaching and learning strategies which promote individual choice we can hinge the future development and progression of our whole profession on a unique methodological approach. Social interaction with students can then be used proactively in formulating their individual plans for achievement across specific aspects of academic curricula, with staff whose expertise underpins the facilitation of core academic principles. As a profession we ought to be committed to building capacity within and between professional groups beyond a tokenistic approach by providing curricula enhanced by real practitioners dealing with real patients, with interprofessional learning at its heart. By developing and nurturing practitioners who are committed to working with one another with the ultimate aim of improving the student experience, we demonstrate the fundamental ability of the profession to care not only about the academic achievement of our students but also their broader contribution to healthcare specifically and the big society generally. By engaging students in the concept of active citizenship, encouraging their contribution to wider society and by giving all curricula encompassing our profession a philosophical underpinning of patient-centred care, we can as a professional body begin to gain the recognition we so richly deserve for producing one of the most diverse arrays of practitioners equipped with the generic capability of working across and between multidisciplinary healthcare teams for the ultimate benefit of the patients we serve.

References

Anderson, L.W. and Krathwohl, D.R. (eds.) (2001). *A Taxonomy for Learning, Teaching, and Assessing: A Revision of Bloom's Taxonomy of Educational Objectives*. New York: Longman.

Brandist, C. (2002). *The Bakhtin Circle: Philosophy, Culture and Politics*. London: Pluto Press.

Colbert, C.Y., Mirkes, C., Cable, C.T., Sibbitt, S.J., Van Zyl, G.O. and Ogden, P.E. (2009). 'The patient panel conference experience: what patients can teach our residents about competency issues' in *Academic Medicine*, **84**(12): 1833–1839.

Cornelissen, E., Mitton, C. and Sheps, S. (2011). 'Knowledge translation in the discourse of professional practice' in *International Journal of Evidence Based Healthcare*, **9**(2):184–188.

Cunningham, D., McCalister, P. and MacVicar, R. (2011). 'Practice-based small group learning: what are the motivations to become and continue as a facilitator? A qualitative study' in *Qualitative Primary Care*, **19**(1): 5–12.

Daniels, H. (2008). *Vygotsky and Research*, Taylor and Francis e-Library.

Dharamsi, S., Ho, A., Spadafora, S.M. and Woollard, R. (2011). 'The physician as health advocate: Translating the quest for social responsibility into medical education and practice' in *Academic Medicine*, **86**(1): 1108–1113.

Eaton, D.M., Redmond, A. and Bax, N. (2011). 'Training healthcare professionals for the future: Internationalism and effective inclusion of global health training' in *Medical Teacher*, **33**(7):562–9.

Jovchelovitch, S. (2007). *Knowledge in Context: Representations, Community and Culture*, Routledge, Taylor and Francis e-Library, 2007.

Juliano, P.J., Black, K.P., Lynch, S.A. and Pradhan, A. (2010). 'Residency Review Committee (RRC) foot and ankle curriculum: we don't need to reinvent the wheel' in *Foot and Ankle International,* **31**(3): 260–263.

Kerno, S.J. (2008). 'Limitations of communities of practice: A consideration of unresolved issues and difficulties in the approach' in *Journal of Leadership and Organisational Studies*, **15**(1): 69–78.

Krathwohl, D.R., Bloom, B.S. and Masia, B.B. (1964). *Taxonomy of Educational Objectives, the classification of educational goals– Handbook II: Affective Domain*. New York: David McKay Co.

Lave, J. and Wenger, E. (1991). *Situated Learning: Legitimate Peripheral Participation*. Cambridge: Cambridge University Press.

Levinson, W. and Pizzo, P.A. (2011). 'Patient-physician communication: it's about time' in *Journal of the American Medical Association*, **305**(17): 1802–1803.

Liu, C.H. and Matthews, R.S. (2005), 'Vygotsky's philosophy: constructivism and its criticisms examined' in *International Education Journal*, **6** (3): 386–399.

Lown, B.A., Kryworuchko, J., Bieber, C., Lillie, D.M., Kelly, C., Berger, B. and Loh, A. (2011). 'Continuing professional development for interprofessional teams supporting patients in healthcare decision making' in *Journal of Interprofessional Care*, **25**(6): 401–408.

Matthews, L.R., Pockett, R.B., Nisbet, G. Thistlethwaite, J.E., Dunston, R., Lee, A. and White, J.F. (2011). 'Building capacity in Australian interprofessional health education: perspectives from key health and higher education stakeholders' in *Australian Health Review*, **35**(2): 136–140.

Neville A.J. (2009). 'Problem-based learning and medical education forty years on. A review of its effects on knowledge and clinical performance' in *Medical Principles and Practice*, **18**(1): 1–9.

Perry, W.G. (1970). *Forms of Intellectual and Ethical Development in the College Years: A Scheme*. New York: Holt, Rinehart and Winston.

Perry, W.G. (1981). 'Cognitive and ethical growth: The making of meaning' in A.W. Chickering and Associates, *The Modern American College*. San Francisco: Jossey-Bass.

Piaget, J. (1950). *The Psychology of Intelligence*. New York: Routledge

Ponsky, J.L. (2004). 'Addressing the "general competencies": what is this all about?' in *Surgery*, **135**(1): 1–3.

Raymond-Seniuk, C. and Profetto-McGrath, J. (2011). 'Can one learn to think critically? – a philosophical exploration' in *Open Nursing Journal*, **5**(1): 45–51.

Rodriguez, H.P., Anastario, M.P., Frankel, R.M., Odigie, E.G., Rogers, W.H., von Glahn, T. and Safran, D.G. (2008). 'Can teaching agenda-setting skills to physicians improve clinical interaction quality? A controlled intervention' in *Medical Education*, **14**(8):3–4.

Symons, A.B., Swanson, A., McGuigan, D., Orrange, S. and Akl, E.A. (2009). 'A tool for self-assessment of communication skills and professionalism in residents' in *Medical Education*, **8**(9):1–3.

Webb, A.R. (2009). 'Emotional intelligence training and evaluation in physicians' in *Journal of the American Medical Association*, **301**(6): 601–603.

Wenger, E. (1998). *Communities of Practice; Learning, Meaning and Identity.* Cambridge: Cambridge University Press.

Westbrook, R.B. (2005). *Democratic Hope: Pragmatism and the Politics of Truth*. Ithaca and London: Cornell University Press.

Williamson, G.R., Callaghan, L., Whittlesea, E., Mutton, L. and Heath, V. (2011). 'Longitudinal evaluation of the impact of placement development teams on student support in clinical practice' in *Open Nursing Journal*, **5**(1): 14–23.

Chapter Seven

Human Factors and Critical Reflexivity in Podiatric Practice

Rob Colclough and Dr Kathryn King

Adverse outcomes

It is accepted that medical interventions are not entirely reliable and can result in harm being done to the patient. This can precipitate litigation and if prosecution is successful, the award of damages. The *Guidelines for the Assessment of General Damages in Personal Injury* (Judicial Studies Board, 2010) provide an established guide for the assessment of damages. For example, if the outcome results in the amputation of a foot then general damages (for pain, suffering and loss of amenity) are typically in the range of £55,000 to £72,000. Additional damages through past and future loss of earning, aids and special equipment, medical costs, patient care and attention, can increase the overall award substantially. In 2010 a man accepted £250,000 in damages from Medway NHS Foundation Trust after a series of failures led to the amputation of one leg and near amputation of the other. The Trust did not admit liability for the failures (www.kentnews.co.uk/news/amputee_accepts_163250_000_compensation_from_nhs_1_1064824 (accessed 07/10/12)).

The practice of podiatry in terms of risks to patient safety and adverse events is notable by the dearth of published serious incidents in the medical and legal literature (Baker *et al.*, 2004; Davis, 2001) and the fact that most errors are not overtly serious. One must assume that podiatry interventions are inherently of minimal risk to the patient with a genuine lack of serious harmful outcomes (Fletcher, 2012).

Alternatively, does this lack of adverse outcomes arise due to factors such as: the highly reliable methods utilised by highly competent practitioners; the rigorous use of safety sciences; the low risk physical environment of podiatric practice; the safety conscious ethos of the practitioners; the quality of clinical governance; a belief that an undesirable outcome could not have been attributable to podiatric intervention … or combinations of these factors (Rogers, 2012)?

It is likely that with the evolution of podiatry into more invasive interventions ('Limitation extended: Hydes vs. East Midland Strategic Health Authority,' 2011), the hazards inherent in those interventions whether they are diagnostic or therapeutic, will pose risks to the safety of patients (Easley, 2005). This chapter explores the theory of combined human and systems fallibility – human factors – in the context of healthcare.

> The human factors approach to adverse events does not position those at the sharp end of the event as sole perpetrator. The human factors approach to adverse events attempts to identify all sources of risk and their contribution to the adverse event.

'Reducing error and influencing behaviour' is the key document in understanding the Health and Safety Executive (HSE) approach to human factors (HSE, 2009). It gives a simple introduction to generic industry guidance on human factors, which it defines as follows:

> *Human factors refer to environmental, organisational and job factors, and human and individual characteristics, which influence behaviour at work in a way which can affect health and safety.*

The Clinical Human Factors Group outline clinical human factors in relation to a clinical setting as follows:

> *Enhancing clinical performance through an understanding of the effects of teamwork, tasks, equipment, workspace, culture, organisation on human behaviour and abilities, and application of that knowledge in clinical settings.*
>
> (The Clinical Human Factors Group, 2011)

Risk assessment and human factors

The recognition of hazards and their associated risk assessment is an accepted standard in clinical and surgical practice and high on the quality assurance agenda in professional organisations. In this context, risk assessment aims at preventing and minimising risk to professional carers and patients alike.

The first step in this process is for the practice or organisation to identify the hazards associated with a particular task or process by referring to the requirements of directives, standards, regulations, good practice and any supplementary information to support the risk assessment process (National Patient Safety Agency, 2009; Lamont, 2012). Deciding who might be harmed by the procedure and how the individual may be harmed and immediate essential care is the next phase.

Legislation requires employers to exercise all reasonable care to protect people from harm. The easiest way to address this third step is to compare your current practice with the requirements of the medical directives and regulations and accepted good practice. Risk reduction (control) measures commence with elimination of the hazard from the workplace altogether; utilising engineering controls to provide optimum working conditions; establishing a policy on user education and a mechanism for reviewing this policy; providing standard operating procedures to provide, if appropriate, step-by-step guidance on a procedure or task; constructing, publicising and frequently reviewing the risk assessment.

Despite preventative measures, there can be a failure in communication or systematic error that can breach the barriers built into the risk assessment. The study of these characteristics has evolved from the field of ergonomics and is called human factors. As applied to healthcare, human factors focus on the working environment, organisational and personal characteristics which influence behaviour (Carthey & Clarke, 2011) and so contribute to providing high quality patient care and safe clinical practice.

What behavioural characteristics lead to adverse patient outcomes? Are such outcomes preventable and how can such an outcome be eliminated in future care? Some of the human factors that contribute to a reduction in patient safety include failure:

- in teamwork and social barriers (Manser, 2009)
- of cognition (e.g. comprehension of instruction)
- of the physical environment

- in the physical demands of the job
- of technological device/product design
- in process/pathway/schedule design.

(Carthey and Clarke, 2011)

Patients expect their provider to alleviate their suffering. For some however the situation can be different. The phrase 'wrong site / side surgery' (Kwaan *et al.*, 2006; New York Times, 1995) typifies a sentinel event that is substantially under the control of humans working at the 'edge of care'.

Beckingsale and Greiss (2011) report a failure of communication between orthopaedic surgeon and patient in the (simple) task of identifying toes. Patients were asked to identify either numerically or descriptively individual digits where there was (a hypothetical) pain. The use of incorrect terminology and the difference between patient and surgeon nomenclature was apparent, particularly on the second and fourth toes of the left foot. The authors recommend the need for the use of unified terminology by the orthopaedic profession when communicating with patients regarding their toes. They suggest a digital nomenclature, like that used in the hand of big, index, middle, ring and little toes for clarity. 93% of all the potential communication errors in this study were due to incorrect use of numbers.

An awareness of these human factors provides a mechanism that can:

- explain why professional practitioners err from established practice
- develop an organisational culture that puts patient safety at the core of clinical practice
- identify potential points where care can be less than optimum and predict what that outcome might be
- enhance and develop the practice of the workforce and the professional body.

Interventions on human factors will not be effective if they consider these aspects in isolation. The scope of what we mean by human factors includes organisational systems and is considerably broader than traditional views of human factors and ergonomics. Human factors should be included within a good safety management system and so can be examined in a similar way to any other risk control system. Human factors and their role in patient safety are fundamental to the ethos of a high quality and trustworthy healthcare provision.

Human factor models and how they contribute to failure of standards of care

Pope's aphorism 'to err is human and to forgive divine' (Pope, 2008) suggests that fallibility is a natural human trait with the corollary that blame should not be apportioned. This philosophy should be embedded into the organisational systems and adopted by all individuals within the organisation. Even in the established methods used in podiatric care, there is always a chance that such care can result in serious consequences for the patient.

Reason (2008) argues that human error can be considered in two ways:

- the 'person approach'
- the 'system approach'.

The models contrast in their approach to human fallibility management.

The 'person approach'

Traditionally, in podiatry as elsewhere, the view is that human errors that result in breaches of patient safety arise from aberrant physiological and psychological processes. These include tiredness, distraction, carelessness and forgetfulness (Sharit, 2006).

Countermeasures utilise legislative techniques to reduce variation in behaviour of the individual by introducing, for example, policies, guidelines, standard operating procedures. Typically doubt is cast on the behaviour of the individual or group, a 'name, blame and shame' approach, with a range of the associated threats that might extend to actual disciplinary action. This provides greater satisfaction for the organisation, it is not behaving irresponsibly, and it has processes that manage these incompetent deviant practitioners.

This personal degradation approach is not the most appropriate mechanism to apply to medical practice (Emanuel *et al.*, 2008; Dekker, 2011). It is thought that personal blaming might slow the progress of safer healthcare organisations by isolating unsafe actions from their system context. The investigative focus is typically on the individual or the group, who is often highly competent.

Adverse events tend to be systematic and don't exhibit non-random patterns. The same circumstances can provoke similar errors with different participants. The desire for enhanced safety is impeded by an approach that fails to address the error-provoking properties inherent within the system.

The military, aviation and engineering industries culturally accept that most mishaps are judged as humanly blameless (Reason, 1997; Marx, 1999). They are described as being '**high reliability**' organisations – they operate in very hazardous circumstances but have fewer adverse outcomes than expected. These high reliability organisations provide best practice models for the healthcare organisation or practitioner.

It is essential that effective management of risk depends upon an overt, blame-free reporting culture that analyses actions and evaluates just where 'the line is to be drawn' and that we recognise it before crossing it (Patankar, 2002).

The 'system approach'

A **system mechanisms approach** acknowledges that humans are indeed imperfect in terms of behavioural traits. Mistakes are seen as consequences, with their source in the fallibility of the system rather than the individual. The solution lies in making changes in the circumstances in which we operate. A central tenet behind the systems approach is to construct a series of safeguards and checks at stages in the process, so that when an error does occur it is the effectiveness of the barrier at that stage which is scrutinised not the individual. The aspiration of the systems approach is to be comprehensive in the recognition of sources and correction of error, inclusive of person, group, the working environment and the organisation.

The aviation industry utilises a system of barriers, often technological, to identify a deteriorating engine or turbine performance and ensure timely amelioration. This is literally, a series of challenging checklists completed by experts often in duplicate. The presence of experts can address whether or not there should be variation from the protocol and the subsequent consequences of that variation will be identified in follow-up checklists. Where there is no fail-safe mechanism, the experts can halt the process or continue. But as a part of the managerial process, there is automatic feedback to the organisation to address the 'blue screen' (or critical error) scenario and additional guidance and training is provided. Increasingly technological systems are being utilised in medical practice (Carayon & Wood, 2010).

The barriers between errors and adverse outcomes are arranged consecutively and have been variously modelled. Hollnagel (2004) described them as a series of dominoes, with the final falling domino precipitating the adverse outcome with a singular or multiple converging 'root causes'. This root cause may be arbitrary as there are often other deeper causes (Dekker, 2011).

Reason (2008) describes them as being like slices of Swiss cheese. The barrier is not intact. A single barrier has many fenestrations. The key is not to allow the holes in subsequent barriers to align. The hazard may pass unrecognised through one barrier, '**latent conditions**', but it will be blocked by the next sequential barrier. Only occasionally do these apertures align to allow the hazard safe passage leading to an adverse event – '**active failures**'.

Latent failures are risky, root cause actions, typically psychomotor and cognitive (Zhang *et al.*, 2002), performed by professionals in direct contact (at the 'sharp end') with the patient. Latent failures arise from strategic decisions that implant failure (the 'holes in the cheese') into a single barrier. These holes can be transient – time pressures, staff short-term absence ('the podiatrist was late'), physical and emotional fatigue, excessive work loading, or permanent – unworkable procedures or design inadequacies. They have the potential to be designed out to reduce risk. They usually have a short-lived effect on integrity of the barriers but can stimulate active failure.

Active failures tend to happen at the 'sharp end'. For example, requesting a local anaesthetic containing lignocaine would be recognised at the next stage when the requirement was for a digital block. Active failures are difficult though not impossible to foresee.

Consider the circumstance of a patient with a plantar metatarsophalangeal joint non-ulcerated pressure lesion. Careful diagnosis led to a prescription and application of a temporary plantar orthoses from a material whose mechanical properties are unknown, where the loading on the material is not addressed, and where the accommodative footwear volume is not known and cannot be controlled. Further, the redistributed pedal forces were not determined and quality of tissue perfusion was not considered. Subsequently, on review, the patient presents with multiple de novo dorsal digital pressure lesions.

These systematic, latent conditions align to give rise to the active error, in this example, the dorsal digital pressure lesions. In this scenario, multiple latent failures align, the alarm bells didn't ring at any stage and the adverse outcome was not predicted.

The reality in clinical settings might be that tried mechanisms of care have worked well in the past with no reported harm arising. In pressure situations where time and availability of expertise is at a premium, professionals will cut corners and create 'work-arounds' sometimes deliberately contravening guidance with a perceived benefit to professional, patient and organisation. Over time this becomes the norm – 'this is our way'. The absence of an adverse event fortifies an antipathy toward the staging mechanisms system particularly if the front line professional does not have ownership of the mechanism.

Latent failure can be identified and remedied before an adverse event arises, by having checklists and flowcharts and expertise on-hand at each stage. A proactive, insightful management would develop the stages and all professional carers would recognise that each stage is not free of hazards. The experts would be required to produce (blame-free) reporting of the scenario and the organisation to reappraise its policy systems (infrastructure, investment, leadership, culture, complexity) and provide further guidance.

'High reliability organisations' and developing a positive safety ethos

Progress in human factors has focused on developing instruments to manage errors by creating damage limitation systems (error management) that can compensate for and contain defects that are akin to those in high reliability organisations (HROs). Researchers have investigated the safety attributes of typical HROs; nuclear power plants, naval vessels and air traffic control organisations.

The challenges facing these establishments are similar. They need to manage complex technologies which, should they fail, could cause catastrophic effects, but can also function normally during periods of very high demand. The principal characteristic required to satisfy these requirements includes an intrinsically dynamic, confident and resourceful philosophy. Schulman (2004) argues that even though there is extreme control over the inputs into HROs, the identical nature of the nuclear material for example, the resilience to change can be adopted in medical practice.

HROs expect the worst and so plan for it. This is difficult to sustain as humans are not habitually uneasy and doubtful. The systems approach in an HRO provides its workforce with timely reminders of potential safety breaches and the tools to help recall so as to make the organisation robust to hazards.

Human variability is seen as an essential quality that enables the high reliability organisations to adapt to diverse circumstances. Weick (1987) describes high reliability as a 'dynamic, non-event'. Safety is maintained by timely human adjustments that bring about the desired outcome without undue applause. The HRO can adapt to abnormal local circumstances where control can shift to the expert-on-the-spot whose role is identified by all colleagues. There is in-built redundancy to the degree that the organisation is inherently preoccupied with searching for, and eliminating, failure. The "what if" scenario is the prevalent ethos. The HRO expects to make errors and so trains its workforce to identify, self-manage and resolve adverse events. The aim in healthcare is to achieve a positive patient safety culture by having an organisation where reporting and learning from error is the norm.

Carthey and Clarke (2011) and Woodward (2004) describe a series of features that help define a medical HRO model. These features are:

- an **open** culture where professionals are happy to raise issues of patient safety
- a **just** culture where those involved in an incident are heard with empathy
- a **reporting** culture where professionals have confidence in, and a clear understanding of, the reporting system
- a **learning** culture where the management and organisation are committed to learn from incidents and fully engage employees with the process
- an **informed** culture where the organisation can demonstrate that it and its workforce have learnt and are able to mitigate against future events.

Reflection and Critical Reflexivity

Across the whole range of healthcare practice practitioners frequently face unique and often challenging situations and they therefore need flexible ways of responding to and learning from these situations. As early as 1984 Benner highlighted the usefulness of exploring critical practice as a way of linking theory to practice and reducing the knowledge gap. Today reflective practice is becoming more important particularly as a significant component for nurse education (Scanlan *et al.*, 2002). Dewing (1990) indicates that reflective practice encourages nurses to actively develop their clinical practice and expertise for the purpose of improving and enhancing patient care.

Reflective practice may be defined as the way in which healthcare professionals learn from experience in order to understand and develop practice. Perhaps one way to define reflective practice is to state that we all learn by our mistakes and reflecting on our actions can help us and others not to make those same mistakes again.

Howatson-Jones (2010) suggests that reflective practice is based on experience and intuitive learning, learning that you may not be aware of at the time. However, bringing this learning into awareness by reflection is an important part of *'developing understanding, skill and competence as a practitioner at any stage'*.

Reflection is not a new concept, Dewey (1933) suggested that reflection was: *'Turning a subject over in the mind.'* Whilst Mead (1934) said: *'The turning back of the experience of the individual upon himself.'* Ghaye and Lillyman (2000) described the reflective process as being a transformative process that can change both the individual and the subsequent actions of that individual.

Ethics, research and maintaining safe practice

Research is required to identify the human factors leading to unsatisfactory outcomes in patient care. An ethical critique and wider methodological critique on the research processes adopted in podiatric practice will be presented as a mechanism by which the concept of human factors can be integrated in translating a theoretical evidence base into practice.

When undertaking research, the use of a reflexive theoretical framework is important to conceptualise the research process. Specific ethical theories provide guidelines and prove extremely useful in highlighting potential problems, offering solutions and generally raising ethical consciousness, with particular reference to beneficence, respect and justice (Flinders, 1992; Sieber, 1992; House, 1990). For example, these strategies serve to ensure that the purpose of all research is explicit, that it offers benefits and causes no harm. Furthermore, they require that the researcher is respectful and knowledgeable; ensures confidentiality and anonymity and also guarantees a secure environment for collected data. Additionally, the healthcare practitioner has the responsibility to ensure protection of respondents' rights, and to maintain a safe research environment.

For example the Nursing and Midwifery Council (NMC) states that:

'You must treat people as individuals and respect their dignity ... you must act as an advocate...you must ensure you gain consent.' (NMC, 2008, p.3)

Specific Ethical Issues

The specific ethical issues of any study relate not only to the respondents, but also to the author, and the researcher. The respective issues will be now be addressed using the framework suggested by Miles and Huberman (1994).

a) Worthiness of the Research

The overall aim of a study is to contribute to existing knowledge and offer additional understanding about a given phenomenon. There is generally a 'felt need' to further develop an understanding of a subject under review in order to increase professional competence. It is envisaged that the findings from a research study should not only inform the author's practice but, in addition, would translate to inform, and enhance, provision generally. The literature review, in a research study, clearly spells out the problem area and generally highlights the rationale for the research study.

b) Competence Boundaries

At the start of any study, the main area of concern centres on the level of competence to undertake the research. Limited experience as a researcher, and the possibility of lack of experience would impinge upon the ability to effectively manage the research study. However, a thorough investigation of the principles of the chosen research methodology together with supervisory sessions will equip the novice researcher and ensure that the study design and implementation are both robust and rigorous.

Data, and the concepts and categories derived from them, are developed from the philosophical stance of the researcher and subsequently this stance will guide the research process. When undertaking a qualitative study, for example, the researcher's interest area may be to explore the perceptions of an individual living with a chronic illness such as type 1 diabetes. The population chosen for study is important to identify. In qualitative research the individual is invited to 'tell their story'.

Reflection on an interview process

The stages of the reflective process may be defined as:

- self awareness
- description
- critical Analysis
- synthesis
- evaluation.

(Adapted from Gibbs, 1988)

Gibbs model of reflection (1988) may be used to demonstrate a reflective account of the interview process, for example:

- Did the researcher conduct the interviews in a purposeful and meaningful way?
- Was the research appropriate?
- Was there any threat to anonymity and confidentiality?
- What learning has taken place?

This model of reflection may also be useful when conducting focus group interviews.

Bailey (1978) suggests the use of an interview guide in order to elicit credible meaningful data. Moreover, the researcher should consider the attention span of the individual and take into consideration their cognitive and linguistic abilities.

A review of the literature regarding the process of conducting interviews when undertaking a qualitative research study allows new learning and further develops researcher competence. For example, Kitzinger (1995) suggests that focus groups are a useful method for both exploring and discussing attitudes, and experiences, related to healthcare practitioners. Moreover, this author highlights that the group membership, consisting of between four and eight people, may be specifically selected for the purpose of the research. Additionally, establishing rapport, maintaining confidentiality and establishing researcher credibility and sensitivity are also crucial to allow the researcher to generate meaningful high quality data.

Benefits, Costs and Reciprocity of the Study Population

Identifying the possible benefits that the respective participants may gain from involvement in the study is important. For each of the participants there may have been feelings of recognition, in terms of being listened to, and of being included as participants in this research study. However the individuals may have felt sufficiently satisfied with having the opportunity to tell their story.

Research Integrity and Quality

Miles and Huberman (1994) suggest that quality relates to goodness, which includes the dependability, credibility and transferability of the research study. A research study conducted with integrity and transparency ensures quality. The design of the research study is important to address both the research aim and the research question. Explicit details of the research process, throughout the study, ensure research rigour.

Koch and Harrington (1998) identify the need to examine self and acknowledge personal position and refer to the 'critical gaze turned towards self' as the reflexive approach which is considered to be an essential criterion for ensuring transparency and achieving rigour in qualitative research. The factual description of the research process for a research study together with a critique of self, provides a clear audit trail and demonstrates achievement of rigour. Reflexivity has been identified as providing demonstrable overwhelming benefit to patient outcomes as well as contributing to developing practitioner knowledge and skill and informing clinical practice (Paget, 2001; Daroszeweski *et al.*, 2004; Gustafsson & Fagerberg 2004).

Conclusion

Human factors are concerned with what people are being asked to do in their workplace (the task and its characteristics), and who is doing it (the individual and their competence). Can they do it repeatedly, and for how long? Is it safe? All of these features are influenced by wider societal concern, particularly the patient voice. There is a need to design healthcare services as the co-product of the interaction between clinicians and patients. These are key attributes of a safe, professional and reliable, trustworthy organisation.

Research, as an important contribution to maintaining safe practice, has also been discussed in this chapter. The collective use of Gibbs Model of Reflection (1988) and the Analytical Framework as suggested by Miles and Huberman (1994) have allowed a comprehensive reflective account of the implementation of research processes underpinning current podiatric practice.

A focused approach to critical reflexivity adds 'trustworthiness, goodness and fit' to the research process. The adoption of ethical principles and the researcher's professional stance throughout the study serve to reduce the risk of harm to all the research participants. Adopting a reflexive approach to all areas of work ensures professional competence, which directly translates to improved clinical outcomes.

References

Bailey, K.D. (1978). *Methods of Social Research*. New York: Free Press.

Baker, G.R., Norton, P.G., Flintoff, V., Blais, R., Brown, A., Cox, J., Etchells, E., Ghali, W.A., Hebert, P., Majumdar, S.R., O'Beirne, M., Palacios-Derflingher, I., Reid, R., Sheps, S. and Tamblyn, R. (2004). 'The Canadian Adverse Events Study: the incidence of adverse events among hospital patients in Canada' in *Canadian Medical Association Journal (CMAJ)* **170**(11): 1678–1686.

Beckingsale, T.B. and Greiss, M.E. (2011). 'Getting off on the wrong foot. Doctor–patient miscommunication: A risk for wrong site surgery' in *Foot and Ankle Surgery*, **17**(3): 201–202.

Benner, P. (1984). *From Novice to Expert: Excellence and Power in Clinical Nursing Practice*. New York: Addison Wesley.

Carayon, P. and Wood, K.E. (2010). 'Patient safety: The role of human factors and systems engineering' in *Studies in Health Technology and Informatics*, **153**: 23–46.

Carthey, J. and Clarke, J. (2011). *The 'how to guide' for implementing human factors in healthcare*. London: Patient Safety First. http://www.patientsafetyfirst.nhs.uk/ashx/Asset.ashx?path=/Intervention-support/Human%20 Factors%20How-to%20Guide%20v1.2.pdf (last accessed 20/06/12).

Clinical Human Factors Group, available at http://www.chfg.org/ (last accessed 20/06/12).

Daroszewski, E.B., Kinser, A.G. and Lloyd, S. I. (2004). 'Socratic method and the internet: using tiered discussion to facilitate understanding in a graduate nursing theory course' in *Nurse Education*, **29**(5): 189– 191.

Davis, P., Lay-Yee, R., Schug, S., Briant, R., Scott, A., Johnson, S. and Bingley, W. (2001). 'Adverse Events Regional Feasibility Study: indicative findings' in *New Zealand Medical Journal*, **114**: 203–205.

Dekker, S. (2011). *Patient Safety: A Human Factors Approach*. Florida USA: CRC Press, Taylor and Francis Group.

Dewey, D. (1933). *How We Think*. Boston: DC Heath & Co.

Dewing, J. (1990). 'Reflective practice' in *Senior Nurse*, **10**(10): 26–28.

Easley, M.E. (2005). 'Medicolegal aspects of foot and ankle surgery' in *Current Orthopaedic Related Research*, **433**: 77–81.

Emanuel, L., Berwick, D., Conway, J., Coombes, J., Hatlie, M., Leape, L., Reason, J., Schyve, P., Vincent, C. and Walton, M. (2008). What exactly is patient safety? in *Advances in Patient Safety: New Directions and Alternative Approaches*, Agency for Healthcare Research and Quality. avalable at: http://www.ahrq.gov/qual/advances2/ (last accessed 20/06/12).

Fletcher, J. (2012) 'Critical event analysis: learning from past mistakes to prevent amputations' in *The Diabetic*

Foot Journal, **15**(3): 112–118.

Flinders, D.J. (1992). 'In search of ethical guidance: Constructing a basis for dialogue' in *Qualitative Studies in Education,* **5**(2): 101–116.

Ghaye, T. and Lillyman, S. (2000). *Reflection: Principles and Practice for Healthcare Professionals.* Dinton: Quay Books/Mark Allen.

Gibbs, G. (1988). *Learning by Doing: A Guide to Teaching and Learning Methods.* Oxford: Oxford Polytechnic Further Education Unit, Oxford Brookes University.

Gustafsson, C. and Fagerberg, I. (2004). 'Reflection, the way to professional development?' in *Journal of Clinical Nursing,* **13**(3): 271–280.

Health and Safety Executive (2009). 'Reducing error and influencing behaviour.' London: HSE. ww.hseni.gov.uk/hsg_48_reducing_error_and_influencing_behaviour.pdf (last accessed 20/06/12).

Hollnagel, E. (2004). *Barriers and Accident Prevention.* Aldershot, Surrey, UK: Ashgate Publishing Co.

House, E.R. (1990). 'An ethics of qualitative field studies' in: E.G. Guba (Ed.) *The Paradigm Dialog,* 158–164. Newbury Park, CA: Sage.

Howatson-Jones, L. (2010). *Reflective Practice in Nursing (Transforming Nursing Practice).* Exeter: Learning Matters.

Judicial Studies Board. (2010). *Guidelines for the Assessment of General Damages in Personal Injury Cases.* Oxford: Oxford University Press.

Kegan, R. and Lahey, L. (2001). *How the Way We Talk Can Change the Way We Work: Seven Languages for Transformation.* San Francisco: Jossey-Bass.

Kitzinger, J. (1995). 'Qualitative Research. Introducing focus groups' in *British Medical Journal,* **311**. 299–302.

Koch, T. and Harrington, A. (1998). 'Reconceptualizing rigour: the case for reflexivity' in *Journal of Advanced Nursing,* **28**(4): 882–890.

Kwaan, M.R., Studdert, D.M., Zinner, M.J., Gwande, A.A. (2006). 'Incidence patterns and prevalence of wrong-site surgery' in *Archives of Surgery,* **141**(4): 353–358.

Lamont, T., Watts, F., Stanley, J., Scarpello, J. and Panesar, S. (2010) 'Reducing risks of tourniquets left on after finger and toe surgery: summary of a safety report from the National Patient Safety Agency'. *British Medical Journal,* published 21 April. Available at: www.bmj.com/content/340/bmj.c1981 (last accessed 05/10/12).

'Limitation extended: Hydes v East Midlands Strategic Health Authority' (2011) (Grimsby County Court, 8/3/2010 – Judge Dowse) in *Clinical Risk,* The Royal Society of Medicine Press Limited, 17: 35–36.

Manser, T. (2009). 'Teamwork and patient safety in dynamic domains of healthcare: a review of the literature' in *Acta Anaesthesiologie Scandinavia,* **53**(2): 143–151.

Marx, D. (1999). *Maintenance Error Causation. Federal Aviation Authority (FAA) Annual Program Summary.* Washington DC USA: Office of Aviation Medicine.

Mead, G.H. (1934). 'Mind, self and society' in *Basics of Qualitative Research: Techniques and Procedures for Developing Grounded Theory* (1998), Eds. A. Strauss and J. Corbin. London: Sage.

Miles, M.B. and Huberman, A.M. (1994). *Qualitative Data Analysis: an Expanded Sourcebook.* 2nd edn. London: Sage.

National Patient Safety Agency; National Reporting and Learning Service (2009). *Rapid Response Report NPSA/2009/RRR007: reducing risks of tourniquets left on after finger and toe surgery.* Available at: http://www.nrls. npsa.nhs.uk/EasySiteWeb/getresource.axd?AssetID=65567 (last accessed 05/10/12).

Nursing and Midwifery Council (2008). *The Code: Standards of Conduct, Performance and Ethics for Nurses and*

Midwives. London: NMC.

Paget, A. (2001). 'Reflective practice and clinical outcomes: practitioners' views on how reflective practice has influenced their clinical practice' in *Journal of Clinical Nursing*, **10**(2): 204–214.

Patankar, M.S. (2002). *Root cause analysis of rule violations by aviation maintenance technicians. Federal Aviation Authority (FAA)*. Washington DC, USA: Office of Aviation Medicine. Available at: http://www.hf.faa.gov/docs/508/docs/maint_product780.pdf (last accessed 22/06/12).

Pope, A. (2008). *The Major Works*. (Rogers, P., ed.) (Oxford World's Classics). Oxford: Oxford University Press.

Reason, J. (1997). *Managing the Risks of Organizational Accidents*. Farnham, Surrey, UK: Ashgate Publishing Co.

Reason, J. (2008). *The Human Contribution: Unsafe Acts, Accidents and Heroic Recoveries*. Farnham, Surrey, UK: Ashgate Publishing Co.

Rogers, L. (2012) 'The bunion "surgeons" who are maiming their patients'. *The Mail Online*, published 03/07/12, available at: www.dailymail.co.uk/health/article-2167882/The-bunion-surgeons-maiming-patients.html (last accessed 05/10/12).

Scanlan, J.M., Udod, S. and Care, W.D. (2002). 'Unravelling the unknowns of reflection in classroom teaching' in *Journal of Advanced Nursing*, **38** (2): 136–143.

Schulman, P.R. (2004). 'General attributes of safe organisations' in *Quality and Safety in Health Care*, **13** (Suppl II): ii39–ii44.

Sharit, J. (2006). 'Human error' in *Handbook of Human Factors and Ergonomics*, G. Salvendry ed. 3rd edn. Hoboken, NJ: John Wiley & Sons.

Sieber, J.E. (1992). *Planning Ethically Responsible Research: A Guide for Students and Internal Review Boards*. Newbury Park, CA: Sage Publications.

Weick, K.E. (1987). 'Organizational culture as a source of high reliability' in *California Management Review*, **29**(2): 112–127.

Woodward, S., Randall, S., Hoey, A. and Bishop, R. (2004). *Seven steps to patient safety. The full reference guide*. UK: National Patient Safety Agency/NHS. http://www.nrls.npsa.nhs.uk/resources/collections/seven-steps-to-patient-safety/?entryid45=59787 (last accessed 22/06/12).

Zhang, J., Patel, V.L. and Johnson, T.R. (2002). 'Medical error: Is the solution medical or cognitive?' in *Journal of American Medical Information Association*, **9** (6) [Suppl, S75 – S77].

Website:

http://www.kentnews.co.uk/news/amputee_accepts_163250_000_compensation_from_nhs_1_1064824 (last accessed 07/10/12).

Index